First Breath, Last Breath

Also by Ma Jaya Sati Bhagavati:

The 11 Karmic Spaces:
Choosing Freedom from the Patterns That Bind You

Deep and Simple Wisdom:
Spiritual Teachings of Ma Jaya Sati Bhagavati

First Breath, Last Breath

Practices to Quiet the Mind and Open the Heart

Ma Jaya Sati Bhagavati

KASHI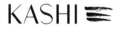

Kashi Publishing
Sebastian, Florida

Published by
Kashi Publishing
11155 Roseland Road
Sebastian, Florida 32958
www.kashi.org

Edited by Swami Matagiri Jaya
Cover and Book Design by Laurie Douglas
Cover Photograph by Swami Dhumavati Jaya
Back Cover Photograph of Ma Jaya Sati Bhagavati by JPI Studios
Photograph of Ma Jaya Sati Bhagavati by Kashi Ashram
Photograph of Neem Karoli Baba by Ramgiri Braun
Drawings by Ma Jaya Sati Bhagavatii

Printed in the United States of America

Before you begin: The benefits attributed to the practices suggested in
this book come from the centuries-old yogic tradition. Results will vary
with individuals. Nothing in this book is to be construed as medical advice.
Please consult a physician before beginning any exercise program.

ISBN-10: 0-9838228-3-2
ISBN-13: 978-0-9838228-3-7

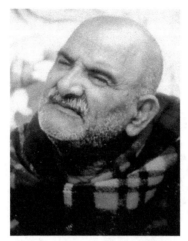

Neem Karoli Baba

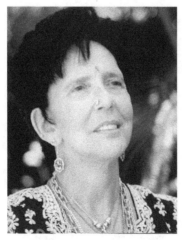

Ma Jaya Sati Bhagavati

The soul breathes beyond time.

Preface

This book is intended as a tool for seekers, with a focus on the ancient practice of *pranayama*, or breath control.

Ma Jaya Sati Bhagavati gave her students hundreds of breath practices. Some she taught in great detail to all of her students; others she gave especially to teachers of her own Kali Natha Yoga system; still others she shared in daily emails.

The editors gathered 200 of these practices, which were given over a 38 year period, 1974 to 2012. We then selected 42 for the present volume. The practices are divided into eleven chapters because many of Ma's teachings involved that sacred number.

The introductions to the breaths are drawn from a wide range of Ma's talks and writings. To share Ma's voice more clearly, we placed a page called "Between Breaths" at the end of every chapter—very lightly edited.

Ma was also a prolific and self-taught artist. The drawings in these pages are hers.

Several of Ma's senior students contributed to developing this book. We realize that it is risky to edit the words of a spiritual genius, yet sometimes it's necessary. We have tried to keep the essence of Ma's words as well as their context. Where we succeed, we are grateful for Ma's continuing guidance. Where we fail, the fault is ours.

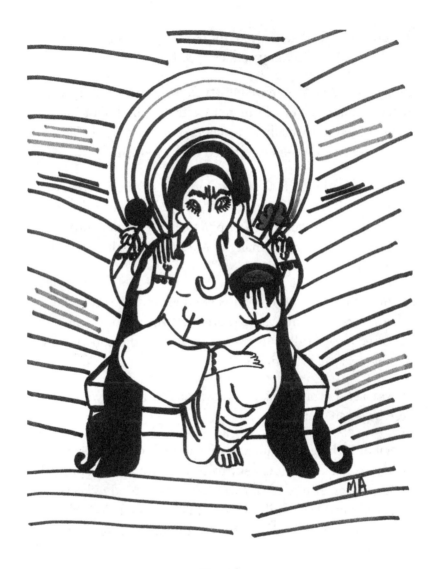

Ganesh

Contents

CHAPTER 1   **The Breath and the Mother** 1

CHAPTER 2   **The Chakras** 7

Ganesh Breath 11

Chakra Meditation 13

The Mother's Heart Cave 15

Between Breaths: The Universal Mother 16

CHAPTER 3   **Opening the Heart** 17

The Vibration of Love 21

The Breath of the Angels 23

The Gift of Completeness 25

An Open Life 27

Break Open the Heart 29

Between Breaths: The Beloved 30

CHAPTER 4   **The Energy of the Universe** 31

Power and Love 35

Greet the Dawn 37

Energy in the Morning 39

Breath of Fire 41

Between Breaths: Mother Kundalini 42

CHAPTER 5   **Giving Up Tension** 43

Release the Shadows 47

Split the Tension 49

Breath of Earth 51

Breath of Space 53

Between Breaths: The Dance of Love 54

CHAPTER 6   **Healing and Healers**...........................55

The Healing Breath of Noticing..............59
Healing Hands.................................61
Aging Beautifully 63
Avoiding Burn-Out: The Chidakash.........65
Between Breaths: No Separation...............66

CHAPTER 7   **Mindfulness and the Moment** 67

Be Still 71
Subtle Awareness.............................73
Simplicity 75
The Mindful Heart 77
Silence.......................................79
Between Breaths: The Moment...................80

CHAPTER 8   **Letting Go**.................................81

Forgiveness 85
The Jasmine Breath 87
Giving Up Fears..............................89
Desire to Be Right 91
Between Breaths: The Black Mother Kali ...92

CHAPTER 9   **Practical Breaths**..........................93

Prayer and Blessing 97
Breath to Lose Weight 99
Conquering Addictions 101
Ending Procrastination 103
Between Breaths: Miracles.....................104

CHAPTER 10   **Ego, Awareness, Intuition** 105

Awareness 109
What Is My Purpose?..........................111
Trust Your Intuition 113
The Sky Mind of the Chidakash 115
Between Breaths: The Inner Universe 116

CONTENTS

CHAPTER 11   **Life, Death, Samadhi** 117

Breath and Non-Breath 121
Breathing with the Dead 123
The Original Thought 125
The River Breath 127
Between Breaths: The River 128

About the Author 131

Glossary 133

CHAPTER ONE

The Breath and the Mother

Your breath is your soul.

In the great spiritual teachings of the world, the mystic has always held the heart of religion. It is the mystic who believes that the moment is deep in wisdom and truth, and we can always be in the moment. When you forget this, or when you doubt yourself, the breath is the tool that will bring you back to awareness.

In this book you will find two types of breath practices. In some, you will use the breath to bring you into a meditative state. In others, you will discover that practicing *pranayama*[1] brings you mastery of the life force through mastery of your breath.

We can distinguish two kinds of life force. First, conscious breathing transforms plain air into *prana*. You can direct and focus prana. There are breaths to bring you energy and breaths to calm you down; there are breaths for the morning and breaths for the night; there are breaths to open your heart or quiet your mind; there are breaths to help you fight addiction or procrastination. There are even breaths to help you lose weight.[2]

The breath can also awaken *kundalini* which is another kind of life force, the feminine force of the universe rising within you.

---

1 Terms are defined in the glossary.

2 Ma Jaya first became aware of the power of the breath when she went to Jack LaLanne's gym in Brooklyn to learn a breathing exercise for weight loss. That breath actually worked for her, and you can find it in Chapter Nine. It also marked the beginning of her awakening.

1

Once awakened, Mother Kundalini transforms your life, doing whatever she must to bring every part of you—body, mind, and spirit—into alignment with the *atman*, or universal consciousness, beyond all dualities. While yoga has many purposes, its highest goal is this profound alignment and awakening. These breath practices are in the lineage of Kali Natha Yoga, also known as Kali Natha Kundalini Tantric Yoga, which embraces this goal.

Kali Natha Yoga is a root yoga which can flower in many ways, both commonplace and profound, depending on the intention of the yogi.

Kundalini *tantric* practices awaken awareness and can lead to experiences of universal energy known as Kundalini Shakti. They offer the possibility of profound transformation.

The word *shakti*, which is used frequently in this book, means the feminine principle of cosmic energy, moving through the entire universe.

The Mother is both inside and outside, and in reality there is no difference. The Mother is the world itself, she is everything you can touch or feel or think, she is illusion, she is reality, she is beauty, she is ugliness, she is everything that has form.

At birth, we are born into the Mother's arms. We come into form, and we take our place within the dimension of space. We are also born into time, and indeed time is the body.

Your whole life, from first breath to last breath, you have the Mother with you in the form of your breath. When you breathe in, the Mother breathes out. When you breathe out, the Mother breathes in.

At death she holds the breath for you, along with all the karma that rides on the breath. When it is time to be reborn, she breathes your own breath into you at the moment of birth.

The universe breathes with you all day, every day, not just at the moments of birth and death.

Everything that has form is constantly changing. There is only one thing certain and unchanging in life, and that is the soul. The individual soul, or *jiva atman*, will eventually merge into the atman, the universal soul. Form will merge with formless, or with what we in the West might call "God the Father." The formless cannot be comprehended by our thoughts of time and space, and cannot be expressed in words. But meanwhile, lifetime after lifetime, it is the breath that allows that soul to be heard on earth. The more you listen to your breath, the more you can hear the voice of your soul.

It is the breath that awakens the Mother to rise within us. Why does she rise? Not to give us worldly power, although that can happen. Not to give us spiritual experiences and visions, although that happens quite often. The Mother's love is there to take us through all the planes of consciousness from lowest to highest, denying nothing.

It doesn't really matter why you start to learn about the breath; when you begin to breathe with awareness, you begin to nourish your self. You also start your journey toward *samadhi*, or profound awareness of God. This awareness is available to all who quiet the mind, and once you begin to know this in the heart core of your being, your life begins to change.

"The heart core of your being?" As you read on, you will hear a lot about the heart. The spiritual heart is in the center of your chest. It is not the physical heart, and it is not the same as the heart chakra, although they are related. The spiritual heart is the seat of the soul, and your true center. As your awareness deepens, you discover that the spiritual heart is the bridge between your personal self and infinity.

To make this real for yourself, before you read too many more words, take three slow deep breaths in and out of the spiritual heart, in the middle of the chest. Visualize the breath coming in horizontally, as if you had an opening there. Feel a warmth in your chest, stay aware of the flow of your breath, and allow yourself to open. This is the start of your journey.

Some of the practices in the pages that follow can be used to improve your everyday life. Others will take you deeper, much deeper, into silence and the moment. Some are widely known among students of yoga and meditation. Others, especially the practices closely identified with Kali Natha Yoga, are known only to a few. In another time and place these might be secrets reserved for advanced initiates, but why hide anything that can bring us closer to our essential selves?

Some of these practices are more powerful than you will realize at first. Take time after you finish any breath or meditation to come back to normal awareness, and don't do anything like driving a car right away. You may find yourself feeling spaced out, or sleepy, or hyper. This will pass.

If you need to return to normal awareness quite quickly, take a few deep breaths into the center of your chest, the spiritual heart. Then rub your palms together vigorously, to bring a heat, and cup them over your eyes. When you're ready, reach up as high as you can with both hands, fingers spread wide, and feel any unused spiritual power flowing out to the universe. This will bring you back into balance. Then *pranam* in front of your heart in gratitude for what you have received. This simple practice will ground you, and you'll be ready to get on with your day.

If you get afraid while doing any of these breaths, just breathe out, open your eyes, and come back to the heart. The body may at times want to gasp for an in-breath, which can add to your fear. There is actually nothing to fear as the breath gets very subtle, or even as it seems to stop. This is your body's preparation for samadhi, and it's as natural as any other physical process. Just remember, you can always breathe out to restart your normal breathing. The out-breath shows you that you actually do have plenty of breath, and you will discover for yourself that the breath knows what to do.

Breath practices are not about straining. If the directions say to hold your breath to a count of sixteen and you find this difficult, you can adjust the timing, and build up gradually. Nobody is judging you, and it's not a contest. You will know when you can push yourself a little more, and when you shouldn't. Of course that goes double if you have a health condition, or if you're pregnant. More specifically, if you are pregnant don't hold the breath for more than a few seconds.

To begin, try a few of these practices, and see where they take you. If you choose a practice that's complicated, just jot down the simplest directions, like how many seconds to hold the breath, and keep those notes near you. Then put the book aside, and begin your journey.

Eventually, your intuition may guide you to a particular practice that you will do daily as part of a regular *sadhana*. Doing any of these breaths consistently for forty days will take you deeper, but that's your choice.

Your posture is a big part of your meditation. Begin by sitting straight and closing your eyes. You don't need to sit cross-legged, but your back should be straight without being stiff. In stillness, there is always fluidity. Gently move your shoulder blades back and down, to help you keep your back straight and prevent you from hunching your shoulders. If you're sitting in a chair, your feet should be flat on the ground. No matter how you sit, take a moment to feel your connection to the earth through your legs and the base of your spine. Then lift your hands, and let them fall in your lap wherever they are comfortable.

Now let your body float, very subtly, just barely moving. Float forward, then to the center; to the left, and to the center; to the right, and to the center; and to the back, and find your center again. This allows your body's own intuition to guide you to the best posture.

Your chin should be just slightly down. Now relax your jaw, and feel your lips touching gently, with the tongue at rest against the upper teeth. Finally become aware of your eyes, look inward, and let the back of your eyes relax. Following these steps, your practice will become easy.

Sometimes the flow of shakti will make you want to nod forward into sleep. Other times, you may feel like gesturing with your hands. Resist both of these impulses. Remember, you want the energy to flow straight up your spine.

Then allow the breath to lead you into the depth of silence. This is your silence, this is your depth; a teacher can lead you to it, but it's yours. The purpose of this book is to offer the tools so you can find your own way.

These are all sacred teachings, to be respected as such, but you know deep down that you deserve to learn them. You will trust yourself more and more as your heart opens more and more. Respect these teachings, use them carefully, and always keep an open heart.

CHAPTER TWO

The Chakras

When Kundalini Mother breaks open a chakra, the light of God enters into it.

We begin our breath practice by learning to recognize the chakras, the energy centers within us. Many people are aware of the seven main chakras, running from the base of spine to the top of the head. There are literally thousands more; for example, there are chakras in our hands and our feet, there are the "blissful chakras" up the side of the rib cage, and there are more chakras above and below the physical body. You can visualize them as wheels of light, always spinning clockwise. It's not quite how they look in most diagrams, though; the main chakras spin horizontally, like hula hoops, from the spinal column around to the front of the body. Energy channels called *nadis* circulate the life forces in the body as the chakras spin, maintaining a balance of divine energy.

The most important upward channel, the *sushumna*, rises inside the spinal column, holding Kundalini. She actually begins to rise from the earth herself, and then through the very tip of the spine, which is sometimes called "the sacred bone." Directly to the left and right of the spine are two more channels. The one that rises from the right, called the *pingala*, carries masculine energy and is associated with the sun; the one that rises on the left, the *ida*, carries feminine energy and is associated with the moon. Or, we might say, the right channel is the soul and the left is the heart.

Mother Kundalini awakens spirituality as she rises through the seven main chakras.

The chakra at the root of the spine is called the *Muladhara*. It is where Mother Kundalini rests until awakened by our awareness. It is associated with the earth.

The second chakra is *Svadhisthana*, in the area of the genitals. It is the source of creativity of every kind, and is associated with the water element.

The *Manipura* chakra is at the level of the navel or solar plexus. This chakra is the home of fire, or power.

Anahata is at the level of the heart and is our center. The heart is vulnerable, and we may fear to open, but we must.

Visuddha, at the throat level, controls how we express ourselves. It is also the gateway to the heart.

Ajna chakra, between the eyebrows, is often referred to as "the third eye." You can learn to see what your earth eyes cannot see.

Finally, the *Sahasrara*, the lotus of 1000 petals, is at the crown of the head. It governs the higher reaches of our being and consciousness. It is said that Shiva and Shakti, the essence of male and female, meet in this chakra and lead us over the head and into different planes of our existence.

Do you need to know all this information on the chakras? Actually, no, you don't. This book is intended as a practical manual, a tool to allow you to feel these things for yourself. You will come to understand the qualities of all chakras as you meditate on them more and more, or as you practice styles of yoga that awaken the spirit as well as the body. You will begin to realize that every chakra affects the actions of our body, mind, and soul, and every action affects the chakras.

Some yogic traditions tell you to stay away from the three "lower" chakras. Instead, greet each chakra like streams from a great river—none less, none more, none higher, none lower. There are no "positive" or "negative" chakras; there are only those that flow freely and those that are stuck. One can be stuck in the third chakra and stay there, focused on power, for lifetime after lifetime. One can also be stuck right under the crown chakra and take lifetimes to move beyond it. Yet if you begin to understand the value of conscious breathing and if you develop a daily practice, you will find that flow. Every chakra can be touched and honored by the breath, and the breath can show you how to flow easily between them.

From the first to the seventh, there is a sacredness to the process. The only danger comes from the forced rising of the Mother Kundalini when the chakras are not ready. This can happen when the heart is closed, or when the whole goal of your practice is to develop power—for example, if you try to hold Kundalini in the second chakra because you think she will strengthen your sexuality, or if you focus only on the third or fifth chakra because you want to gain power over others, or even if you put all your attention on the sixth chakra because you have been lured by the promise of psychic powers. Your fourth chakra, your heart chakra, is where your journey begins and ends. If you make your home in the heart, there really is no danger.

Ganesh Breath

In Hindu tradition, Ganesh is associated with the first chakra and a new beginning. He is known as the remover of all obstacles, and he is often invoked at the start of something new.

As Mother Kundalini rises, Ganesh goes first to clear her path.

In this breath practice, you intentionally release old thoughts and emotions, feelings of unworthiness, or anything that is an obstacle to your inner joy. This leaves space for something new to happen in your life.

Ganesh Breath

Begin by sitting in a comfortable position and place your awareness on your breath coming in and going out. Breathe normally, but let your focus settle softly in your heart.

With every out-breath, visualize any obstacle leaving you. With every in-breath, see a new way of doing things with awareness and vitality.

Continue to watch as problems and limitations arise, and then watch them leave. Practice this for a few minutes.

Now, take a deep breath in to your heart and hold it for a count of 9, and exhale slowly.

Again breathe in, hold for 9, and release slowly. Do this for eleven breaths.

After completing your last breath, just sit quietly for a few minutes breathing normally before rising from your seat to move forward into your day.

Chakra Meditation *When working with the chakras and the breath, the basic pattern is the same: Begin by breathing into the heart; breathe through other chakras as if they were steps on your journey; and return to your heart. This can be a beginning to an awakened life, a life with awareness of the spirit of love, both inside and out.*

This pattern is expressed in many ways, sometimes including additional chakras both above and below the physical body.

When you discover the inner world, your whole existence is put into play and you begin to understand how the Mother lives within you.

We begin with a simple chakra meditation. Begin by breathing in and out of your spiritual heart, the center of your chest, with deep awareness. After establishing a regular rhythm, let yourself fall into the beauty of the breath as you bring it to each chakra. You will breathe in and out of each chakra three times, and then seven times in the highest chakra at the top of your head.

Chakra Meditation

Bring your awareness to the center of your chest, your spiritual heart, and feel the flow of your breath.

Then bring your awareness to the base of your spine, your first chakra, and breathe in and out three times, connecting to Mother Earth. Feel stable, grounded, and nourished.

Bring your awareness to the second chakra, the sexual organs, the place of creativity, movement, and change. Breathe in and out three times.

Focus your attention in the belly, the third chakra, related to the element of fire. Breathe in and out more deeply, fanning this internal fire of transformation.

Rise up now into your heart chakra, and feel your breath as a flow of compassion, love, and gratitude.

Bring your breath up into the throat chakra, the home of communication and creative expression. Feel your throat softening and relaxing.

The sixth chakra, between the brows, relates to light, intuition, and insight. Be very still as you breathe in and out, keeping an inward gaze. Listen to your higher spiritual self within this place of stillness.

At the seventh chakra at the top of your head, visualize breath flowing in and out through the top of your head where the baby's soft spot is. Take seven deep breaths here and feel at peace.

Then gently and slowly bring your awareness back to the center of your chest, and breathe in and out deeply and fully for a few minutes. Experience a new awareness of your breath and your chakras along your spine.

The Mother's Heart Cave *After you practice the more complex breaths, it will become easier to quickly shift your awareness.*

This breath is very simple; you can do it at the start of meditation, or you can do it whenever you want to open your heart.

This breath can become your refuge. It gives you a way to simply rest in your spiritual heart whenever you need to.

The Mother's Heart Cave

Sit quietly, focused on your heart.

Start breathing in to the count of 7, holding the breath for 7, breathing out for 7, and holding the breath out for 7.

Do this sequence at least five times.

Then let the breath become normal.

Be still and keep the focus deep in your heart chakra.

You have entered the cave of the heart, which is the seat of your soul. Feel the Mother who dwells there in her heart cave in the center of your chest.

BETWEEN BREATHS

The Universal Mother

The great Mother is the Mother of all powers. She is the shakti in me and the shakti in you, and she is the shakti of all gods and goddesses. She is the supreme deity of deities.

She is the bestower of the three sources of time, yesterday, today, and tomorrow.

She is the indweller who lives in our hearts. She is the destroyer of all that is negative.

She is the non-dual goddess who, by the power of her maya, can rid you of delusion, the delusion that the ego mind sends all time long.

They who know the Mother who is without beginning or end know the fullness of their own heart chakra and the pure heart of the universe. She is the knower of all, and because she lives within your being, she makes you the knower who has not awoken yet, but who will in time.

We will regulate the breath together. Nothing will be too hard or too easy. Each breath will flow into another. As the moon shines forth and the clouds disperse, you will find you, and you will find me. As the radiant sun reveals itself and scatters darkness, so the darkness that you have been carrying will fall apart and you will welcome pure magnificent light.

You are the keeper, and you are the light. The light who is the Mother sings, dances, smiles, laughs, and shouts with joy. "I am here," cries out the universal Mother. "I am here never to leave you ever, ever, ever."

CHAPTER THREE

Opening the Heart

The power of shakti, which moves the universe, is love.

The spiritual heart is in the center of your chest, to the right of your physical heart. Any time during the day or night, you can focus your breath in the heart and release the knots that have been holding you—knots formed of anger, jealousy, fear, so many things that keep you bound to your small self. An open heart develops an open life.

It sounds simple, and indeed it is, but the ego mind will fight hard to keep control, which often means keeping your heart partly closed. Instead of doing battle with your mind, you can move your attention to a deliberate thought of love. This is not the same as denying any part of your life. Yes, you have pain, and yes, you have negative emotions, but you can refuse to let them run your life. Instead, you can place your attention on your breath, focused in the heart chakra.

Many of us have a wounded heart, still suffering from whatever pain has come to us in the course of our lives. At times it is hard to allow the breath into the wounded heart, yet this is the place that you must bring your attention. As the spiritual heart opens, the scars open too. Or, another way to put it, the expanding spiritual heart pushes out against the crust of fear and negativity that surrounds it. Once you realize that you are loved, you begin to break through the crust that surrounds the spiritual heart. This crust is a shield you have put up. After being hurt, you build a wall of distrust. You think you are safe, but inside your heart is dying a little because you miss who you are. You lose the ability to love yourself. You allow yourself to feel less. You think you are keeping the ego out, when in fact you are sharing a space with the ego when you lock yourself in this place. The poet Rumi used the word "Beloved" to describe spiritual experiences that are not bound by any one religion:

When you find yourself with the Beloved, embracing for one breath,
In that moment you will find your true destiny.

This essence of the Beloved is a powerful feeling that ignites a spark, a passion, a yearning. That spark is the spiritual force that blesses us along the journey. For some it comes in the form of a deity, a teacher, a guru; for many, it is Christ. For others, the Beloved can simply be Nature herself, or the smile in a child's eyes. As each of us is different, so our Beloved is different, and our path is different.

Maybe when you think of love you think of a specific person — your partner, or your child. Yes, but you can also learn to look beyond anything impermanent; all human relationships change no matter how much we want them to go on forever. The Beloved walks through life with you and then meets you again in death. No separation.

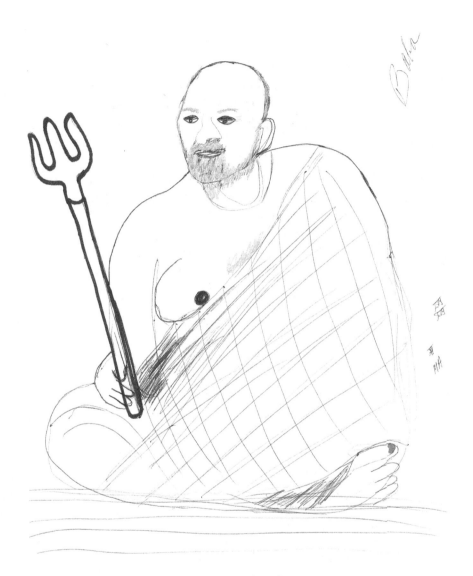

Neem Karoli Baba

The Vibration of Love

In the middle of a busy and stressful day, you may feel you just need to get away for a moment, but often this means distracting yourself by checking your email or having a snack. Instead, try using the breath to take you back to your heart.

This breath is simple, and can be done in ten minutes. If you do it several times throughout the day, you will find yourself living more and more in the vibration of love.

The Vibration of Love

Sit quietly. Close your eyes.

Focus on your spiritual heart in the middle of your chest. Feel your breath, moving in and out of your heart.

Bring your hands together in a tight pranam in front of your fourth chakra. As you breathe, press your hands together and focus on both the third eye and the crown chakra. Feel the third eye and the top of the head open.

Concentrate over the head for a little while and then come back to your heart.

Relax your hands. Sit and meditate in the cave of your heart for ten minutes.

Then breathe in and out slowly five times.

Sit quietly for another five minutes, letting the breath relax and become normal.

Pranam again, and bow to your Beloved.

The Breath of the Angels
Many practices depend on visualization. You can learn to "see" your chakras, you can discover the light that is always with you, and you can learn to use that light to benefit yourself and others. For some, visualization is easy; for others, it is harder and you may feel you are just making things up. Yet visualization is a powerful tool for awakening, a tool known to mystics and yogis all over the world.

How you focus your visualizations is up to you. Although the next practice is called "Breath of the Angels," you don't need to believe in angels. You could just visualize light if the idea of angels doesn't work for you.

Actually you don't need to believe in anything at all except your own beauty; to understand that, you need to open your heart.

The Breath of the Angels

Bring your attention to your heart chakra, feeling a great energy and visualizing a bright light there as you breathe in and out.

Then, with your mind's eye, follow this light as it flows to the right, around your back, and returns to the center of your chest.

When you complete the circle, let the breath out. Feel the light riding on the breath. Leave the breath out, and feel the angels dancing on the tip of the out-breath.

Breathe in light, hold it, and this time visualize it going counter-clockwise (to the left). When you return to the center of your chest, let the breath out, and again feel the angels riding the breath.

Keep doing this, changing the direction of the light each time you breathe in.

If you are doing this during the day or morning, do two extra contractions of the belly at the end of the out-breath. In other words, after you breathe out, breathe out two more short breaths. Then breathe in and start your day. You will feel a surge of energy and shakti.

If you are doing this in the night, then end by just sitting still, being aware of the softness of the breath. Or lie down, knowing that the angels are right there to protect and love you through the night.

Your Beloved is with you on the in-breath and on the out-breath and in the place of no breath at all.

The Gift of Completeness *Affirmations work much the same way as visualizations, in the sense that you don't have to actually believe what you are affirming for it to be effective. You can affirm something like "I am love," even if you don't really think you are. Deep down, at the soul level, you actually* are *love. Gradually this statement will become more of a reality as it helps you connect to the love that lives in your deeper self.*

This is important because people on a spiritual path are hungry to know their true beauty, and so they may feel that they are somehow incomplete. Spiritual hunger can turn into unworthiness, or the feeling that you are just not good enough.

Thoughts of unworthiness infect the body and close the heart, and so they prevent you from feeling the shakti that you need on a spiritual path. To be able to receive the shakti of the Mother and use it in the fullest way possible, you must conquer the deep feeling of unworthiness.

Here is an example of how to use an affirmation with the breath.

The Gift of Completeness

Breathe in through the top of the head and feel the breath drop to the middle of the chest. Meanwhile, internally say these words with a deep conviction: "I am complete within myself just the way I am."

Continue to say these words while you are holding your breath. Hold as long as comfortable. Don't strain.

Let the breath go out, horizontally, from the heart. As the breath goes out, say, "I am complete, I am complete."

Keep breathing in through the top of your head and out through your heart. Do this over and over until your heart tells you to stop.

An Open Life *Neem Karoli Baba asked us to "Feed everyone." He meant food for the body, as well as food for the spirit. In his presence, everything was* prasad, *or blessed food. Your own breath, when you have deep awareness, is also* prasad.

An extended meditation retreat can deepen your spiritual life, but most of us can't withdraw from the world for very long. Even if we could, the goal of spiritual life isn't merely to expand our own consciousness. What will you do with your newfound awareness?

In the end, we will want to feed the world, although that means something different to each of us. Some will focus on nourishing their own families, while others will take a wider view. It doesn't matter what form your service takes, just so long as you follow your heart.

Using the breath, you can refresh your heart quite quickly, and then open your heart to others.

Opening the heart will bring you into a more open life.

An Open Life

Breathe in more deeply than you have ever breathed before.

Send the out-breath as a blessing to someone you resent or dislike.

Oh, you don't want to do this?

Would you really choose to keep those thoughts of revenge or jealousy? Do you want to hold on to pain? NO!

Let it go, and send out a beautiful breath filled with love and hope and joy to someone you dislike.

Now breathe in love deeply and fully. And again send it out to that person.

Keep the breath out for as long as you can, and then breathe in all the breath that you can hold, knowing that the breath comes from the Mother's own heart.

Hold the breath. Feel it spread all around your heart.

Now breathe out as a blessing to someone you love.

Because you have opened your heart without judgment, and because you have not let your negative feelings put limits on love, you may feel more joy in giving than if you refused to bless the one you do not like.

Break Open the Heart

Sometimes as the spiritual heart opens, you may feel emotional pain. To understand this, imagine for a moment that life has placed a hard crust around your heart, keeping it partly closed. So if tears come as you open your heart, it may be that you are pushing against that old crust, cracking it open, making room for love.

For this next practice, keep concentrating on your breath in your heart. If tears come, allow them. It is just your heart opening wider. You are opening up more space in your spiritual heart for the breath of pure love.

Just keep letting go. You will find that after a while you will be able to breathe more deeply than ever before, and you will have more energy.

Break Open the Heart

Sit in a comfortable position and bring your hands to pranam. Explore with your thumbs that sensitive spot in the middle of your chest. Keep your attention right at the sternum, just under that bone. This is your spiritual heart.

You may feel a heaviness there. Perhaps it is an ancient pain. Don't try to understand it, just feel it. Is there sadness? Do you feel fear?

Begin to press gently on that sensitive spot, feeling more and more of the sadness or fear breaking and melting away. You may feel a very noticeable ache or discomfort there. This is a pain born of the losses and fears and tensions of lifetimes.

As you go deeper inside yourself, do not try to protect the heart; let it be open and vulnerable.

In this vulnerable space, understand how deeply the Mother loves you.

Surrender into the feelings. Let the chest open wide. Don't let fear stop you, and don't judge yourself. Just experience all feelings, knowing that the Mother is with you. Let your breath bring you to a soft awareness of love.

Lower your hands and softly breathe in and out of your heart. Sit quietly and enjoy the openness of the heart space.

BETWEEN BREATHS

The Beloved

When you feel that your world is falling apart, or when you feel you are fighting the world and losing, breathe in and know you are not alone.

Your strength will double itself, and more. You will begin to understand that your breath is your Beloved and you are your Beloved's breath.

She is your breath; feel your breath.
She is your heartbeat; feel your heart beating.
She is your mind; feel your thoughts thinking.

Say the name of your Beloved on the out-breath and on the in-breath. This is your thought, your deliberate thought, your chosen thought, not the thought your ego wants to send you.

Begin reaching with your heart for all you need in life.
Reach slowly.
Reach gently.
Breathe.

Breathing with your Beloved allows you to reach anything you need. It brings you into the moment of accepting your own beauty.

Feel the freedom of the breath this moment, even as you read. You are the Mother's breath.

CHAPTER FOUR

The Energy of the Universe

Breath with awareness is prana. Breath without awareness is just air.

We breathe unconsciously, taking the breath for granted each day. Yet the most powerful source of life is your breath, the breath of the universe that is in you. If you make a habit to begin and end your day with five deep breaths, you can change your life.

When your level of energy has fallen, you only need to breathe in deeply from the universe, hold the breath, and feel the shakti flowing through you as you let the breath out. There is an abundance of prana for everyone.

Take a breath right now and hold it, then let it out. Watch the breath going out and into the universe. This is pure prana, the consciousness of the living breath. As you practice and become more aware, allow the out-breath to be slightly longer than the in-breath.

You are breathing with the universe and the Earth. When you realize this, your practice becomes a joy, not a chore, not boring; it is how you nourish yourself. It is when you realize that the Self is none other than the Mother.

Do you fear your own power? Many people do, and so they hide their own greatness not only from the world, but even from themselves. Now, as you read, you can visualize a great white light pouring through your seventh chakra at the top of the head, then down to between your brows, then your throat, and then your heart. Let the light fill every chakra. The light belongs to all of us. By understanding your heritage of light, space, sound, and so much more, you bring to yourself a great amount of divine shakti that was always yours in the first place. Learn to accept it; it is your own shakti and your own beauty.

Or do you love power, maybe a little too much? Many of the breaths that follow will ask you to focus on the third chakra, the place of power. Is this dangerous? It can be, if you misuse power or if you forget where it comes from.

Teachers and yogis often say that the third chakra is the seat of power, and the fourth chakra, surrounding the spiritual heart, is the seat of love. In reality, though, the heart is the true power of the third chakra. As you feed your heart with thoughts and actions of love, nourishment drips into the solar plexus and then falls to the base of the spine and begins to rise up until it reaches the top of the head.

If you ignore the heart and just use power without love, you may find success in the world, but that is all. Power without love is dry and hard, and it brings pain in life. Shakti is the combination of power and love, together. That is why, when you awaken the power of the third chakra, you must have a full and open heart center. The power of the third chakra must always be merged with the heart. Power with love becomes shakti, and then it becomes love supreme.

No matter where your meditations or spiritual exercises take you, always return to the heart. Breathe slowly into the heart for a few minutes, feeling a gentle warmth. Grounded in your heart, you will not abuse your power.

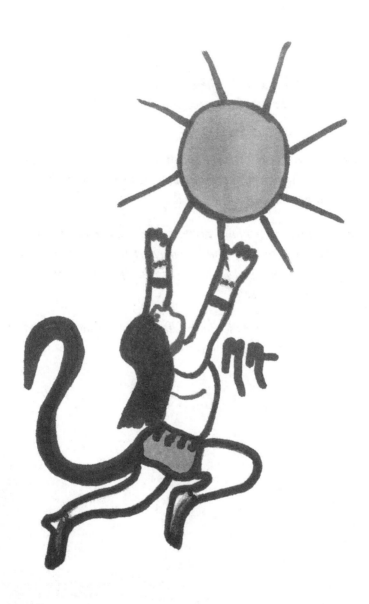

Hanuman

Power and Love *There is a deep and wonderful fire in the third chakra that can give you both worldly power and spiritual power.*

This chakra helps you to take spiritual teachings and bring them into action. The power of compassion begins to be born here, and the strength to fight injustice takes hold.

Treat the third chakra with respect; you could choose to use its power in a negative way and become destructive to yourself and others. That doesn't mean you need to fear power, but you need to be careful not to abuse it.

Always begin your practice with a few breaths into the heart, and return to the heart when you are finished.

Power and Love

Sit and concentrate on your third chakra. Your focus brings
a warmth, awakening a fire that you will be able to direct to
any chakra.

Breathe in to the third chakra. Feel the heat of spiritual power.

Breathe out, and feel the force of the Mother.

Keep your mind on the flame. Let it burn away stale thoughts.

Breathe in and out of the third chakra for eleven minutes.

When you are done, breathe in and out of your heart to restore
your balance.

Remember, power without love is nothing, but opening the
third and fourth chakras together brings a powerful love.

Shakti is the combination of power and love.

Greet the Dawn *A lack of energy and depression reinforce each other. For many of us, depression comes in the morning, as we awaken and think, "Just another day." And so we go through the day not fully awake, buried in negative thoughts, and tired before we even begin.*

This breath invites you to renew your energy before you start a downward spiral into depression.

Greet the Dawn

This morning feel your breath coming into the heart, and the heart expanding, and your breath going out. Feel this, but at first do not try to control the breath.

Now bring your breath deeper into the heart, greeting the new dawn.

Hold your breath in the heart for the count of 7.

Without breathing out, breathe in more. This time breathe directly into your belly, the space of the third chakra, and the seat of power.

Hold for the count of 3.

Then let your breath slowly out of the top of the head, and start again.

Repeat this cycle as long as you have time for.

Feel how this double breath can help you start your day.

Energy in the Morning *When the mind gets polluted*
with things of the world, then the prana becomes cloudy and
impure. The next breath can burn away any impure or stale breath.

Morning meditation allows you to become aware of the shakti
flowing through you in the form of light. When you feel yourself
embraced by dawn's golden orb of light, you are living and
breathing spiritual time, which is timeless.

This is a good breath for the morning, but in reality you can do it
any time throughout the day when you need more energy.

Energy in the Morning[3]

Breathe in for the count of 4.

Hold the breath for the count of 16.

Then breathe out for the count of 8. Hold the breath out for the count of 8, and start over.

Do this sequence five times.

Then breathe in for the count of 5.

Force the breath out strongly for the count of 5.

Do this sequence five times.

Then let the breath do what it will, and feel the shakti you have brought to your morning.

---

3 If you struggle with the suggested counts, feel free to adjust them, but keep the same ratio. So, instead of 4-16-8-8, you might start with 2-8-4-4.

Breath of Fire *As you go through your day, you may feel yourself losing energy and focus. Breath of fire,* or Kapalabhati, *stimulates the area of the third chakra, which regulates our health and vitality. Just a few seconds of the fire breath can help you get your energy back.*

Breath of fire is integrated into many of the asanas in Kali Natha Yoga, and is done while you hold a pose. If you're not with a qualified teacher, just do it while you sit straight and tall, keeping your shoulders and spine steady.

Fire breath is not recommended if you are pregnant. However, it can help with the hot flashes that come with menopause! You don't need more heat, obviously, but it can balance out the heat you are feeling. In this case, do your fire breath slowly and steadily.

Breath of Fire

Settle yourself into a comfortable sitting position, with a straight back.

Take a deep breath in to your belly, and let it about halfway out.

Then begin to exhale quickly and sharply, again and again. Use the muscles of your lower abdomen to push the breath out.

The in-breath will automatically take care of itself, while you stay focused on the powerful out-breath. The only part of your body that should move is your belly. Keep your back steady.

You can do a fire breath slowly and powerfully, as if you are awakening a smoldering flame. Or, you can do it quickly, fanning the flame to reach higher. One breath per second is a good steady speed that you can maintain.

Don't overdo this. Start with just fifteen seconds, and don't do more than a minute at a time.

BETWEEN BREATHS

Mother Kundalini

Mother Kundalini, or "serpent power," is the life force of the universe within us. When the serpent is asleep and curled three and a half times at the base of the spine, the world is covered in ego. As soon as you look up and welcome awareness, she uncurls and rises through the divine wheels that begin to spin in great joy.

She brings to her children the potential to grow with the creative force of the universe, which is beyond the human mind or the ego's thoughts. Her presence permeates thought.

As Mother Kundalini rises, thousands of karmas lose their strength to keep you bound. The bondage of negativity becomes worn.

She is the indweller of all. She is the inner sound of the nothingness.

The path where she leads you is pure bliss. It is the path of love and peace. It is the path of shakti and calmness.

She creates stepping-stones with all that you have learned from your mistakes.

The conscious expansion we feel when Mother rises is tremendous. It awakens us. The lotuses open wide and bubble with joy. They burst into love. All is known.

Open to the call of the Mother. Dance with her as she rises toward Lord Shiva.

CHAPTER FIVE

Giving Up Tension

You do not need tension to understand life.

The breath is the essential energy of life. Bringing yourself more prana can give you great energy, but it can also help you relax and flow with the currents of life.

When you let life upset you, the jagged edge of your emotions touches everything. You may not even remember what it is that upset you in the first place as you let little things grow big and take your life force from you. This blocks your deep intuition and causes you to leave your center.

Whenever you come across a tense moment, just begin to pay attention to your breath and watch it slow down. As the breath gets slower, you will feel yourself becoming calmer and more relaxed. You will find that you will be more in your heart and you will be able to handle situations better. You will begin to engage the heart more and more, leaving the ego mind behind.

Your breath will become your sanctuary.

Deep tension gathers not only in your muscles, but also in your chakras, where it blocks the free flow of energy. As you do any calming practice, concentrate not on the tension itself, but on the shakti that is gathering in your body.

Breathe deeply whenever you can remember. Just by taking a few minutes in the middle of your day, you will be amazed how calm you will become. You are always in the light of love, but you may not be aware of it. You can find a comfortable space inside of you that you can return to time after time.

Every mystic knows that the true journey is inward. With the lessening of stress, it is easier to find your spirit, which truly is your essential self. There is no tension in the soul. No words are needed, no thoughts are required, only love.

And yet, we need some practices to help us dissolve our old habits of stress and tension, old habits that have taken root in the body as well as the mind. Some of it is stale tension, which you can carry with you from lifetime to lifetime. This is karmic tension, far deeper than the stress of daily living. You can't let go of all your stale tension at once, but you can practice letting go bit by bit with these practices.

When you are breathing in and expanding your lungs and chest, know that the universe is breathing into you and breathing out of you. You are doing nothing but allowing the universe to do its job. Thus you can relax. You are in control of your own life, and yet in a deeper way it is the universe that is in control.

How small your tension becomes when you remember who you really are!

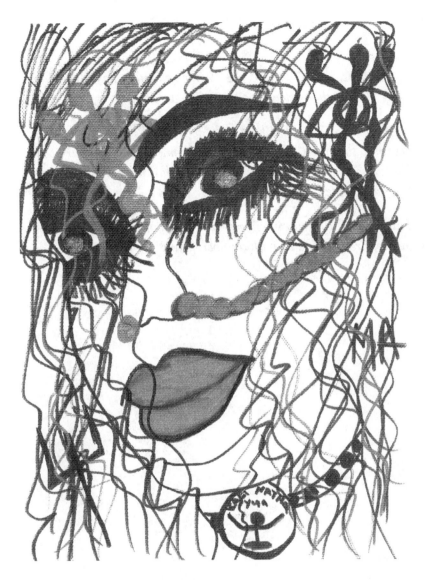

Bhagavati

Release the Shadows *We begin with a basic method of using the breath to release pain, tension, or anxiety.*

Begin with awareness. Where is the tension? When you bring the breath to that area, you can give up chronic tension in your body. You can also loosen the stale tension that has taken root in your body as an effect of karma.

This is breathing with intention—the intention of becoming an aware, stress-free being with an open heart!

Release the Shadows

Scan your body for any stress or anxiety, and let the tension go on the out-breath. You can feel the stress leaving like a shadow that comes into the light and disappears in the brightness.

Now begin to direct the in-breath to where there is stress, and slowly let it out. Do this for at least fifteen minutes, feeling the staleness leave your body.

Then just sit and let the breath do what it may.

If you are going to sleep, breathe in slowly and breathe out ever so slowly, and lie down with the Mother's arms wrapped around you.

If you are starting your day, end by doing the fire breath[4] for a little while. Then take at least one deep breath into the heart.

---

4   Breath of fire is explained on p. 40-41.

Split the Tension
When growth is restricted, it is easy for the ego to send us thoughts of sadness and depression. The ego mind doesn't like to give up stress. Constriction is the ego's friend, but you are not your ego, and you can take charge of your life.

With the next breath, you are literally breaking up the tension into smaller pieces, and letting go of some of them. Once the tension is split, it has no power. It will finally fall apart and disappear.

Is this too simple to be believed? You don't have to believe, just try it for yourself.

Start your day with this breath or do it any time when you get a few moments alone. Do it as much as you want over a period of days or weeks, until there is very little tension, just a calm response to whatever is going on in your life.

Split the Tension

Take a deep breath, sit quietly, and deliberately tense the whole body. When you are fully conscious of this tension, release it completely with a big sigh on the out-breath, and just become like a rag doll.

Repeatedly tensing and letting go will allow your blood to circulate and prana to flow freely. You start to loosen up.

Next, sit quietly, with a straight back. Breathe in and out of each chakra one time, starting from the base of the spine. Visualize the breath flowing in and out horizontally. This is an easy natural breath. Do not strain.

Just notice, which chakra feels clogged? For instance, if you are holding a lot of anger, the blockage might be in your third chakra, the seat of power.

You have gone through all your chakras once; now return to the base of the spine and start again. This time make an effort to breathe deeper and more fully than before.

Soon you will reach the chakra you chose to focus on. When you get there, breathe in and out of that chakra 4 times, horizontally.

The fifth time you breathe into the blocked chakra, send the breath gently out of the top of the head, visualizing the upward flow. Meanwhile say to yourself, "Split the tension, split the tension…." Keep saying it over and over as you breathe out slowly.

Staying in the chakra you have chosen to focus on, keep breathing in horizontally, and breathing out as an upward flow through the top of the head. As you breathe out, say to yourself, "The tension is split, the tension is split…."

Breath of Earth *Most of the breaths in this chapter involve releasing tension or negativity through the out-breath from your seven main chakras. But there are many chakras, including important ones in your feet.*

As is often said in Tai Chi and similar disciplines, "You stand between heaven and earth." This is true, whether you stand, sit, or kneel, whether you wear shoes or go barefoot, and even if you are on a high floor of a tall building. Mother Earth holds you.

The next breath will help you remember that.

Breath of Earth

Sit on a chair with your feet flat on the floor.[5] Become very aware of your contact with the earth. Watch closely and feel your natural breath coming in and out, without trying to change it.

After a little while, begin to make the out-breath a little longer than the in-breath.

Being aware of the bottom of your feet, feel that all your stress is draining out of you into the earth.

When a lot of the tension is gone, you can discover a healing source of shakti that comes into the soles of your feet. At first it may feel strange, yet nevertheless it feels good—no, it feels great.

Pay little or no attention to any of your thoughts.

Remember to say, "It is just a thought, it is just a thought…." Actually see the thoughts in a clear bubble. The bubble pops, and the thoughts just drift away, hurting no one, especially yourself. You are just here, on the earth.

Sit for a few minutes more. End your meditation with a focus on your heart, and feel a flow of love entering through your chest.

---

5   You can also do this breath while lying flat on your back. Just be very aware of the earth beneath you.

Breath of Space *Behind your upper front teeth there is
a fleshy ridge. When you press your tongue against this ridge and
breathe out, tension and staleness are leaving your body. You are
actually performing a* mudra, *a ritual gesture or energetic seal. This
mudra settles the body and brings balance, and you can use it at
times of stress and confusion.*

*When doing breath practices, we sometimes get afraid. We may
feel as if we will run out of breath. With staleness gone, you will
discover that you have enough inner space and enough breath, and
you can let go of fear.*

Breath of Space

Close your eyes and gently press the tongue onto the ridge behind the upper front teeth.

With the mouth slightly open, breathe out completely. You are creating open space within, as tension and staleness leave you.

Keeping the tongue in place, close the mouth, inhale to the count of 4.

Hold for the count of 7.

Slowly breathe out, mouth slightly open, for the count of 8, keeping the tongue behind the upper front teeth.

Close the mouth; hold out for the count of 4.

Now, take a few resting breaths, and see how you feel. Do you sense that you have opened up more inner space?

Begin this sequence again, starting with an exhale.

BETWEEN BREATHS

The Dance of Love

Woven into the heart of every human being is the dance of love.

It lives in the inner world of our being. It does not belong to the time or the space of life or death. It is always there just behind the curtain of existence.

It is like a fragrant scent; it is invisible, yet it is present. It is neither in this world or another. It permeates both.

This dance is not brittle nor can it be stopped, yet deep in the shadows of ego one can find it hard to hear the music of the dance.

To find your true quiet self, watch your breath coming in and out. Ride on the wings of your breath into the dance of life.

CHAPTER SIX

Healing and Healers

There is no prayer greater than service.

The fastest way to God is the road of service. Yes, you need silence, you need meditation, you need prayer, but along with all that you need to open your hands to create a healing space, to touch, to comfort, or to build. The more you live your life from a place that is not driven by your small ego, the freer you become. This happens especially when you forget yourself in taking care of someone else.

You have heard the phrase "selfless service." Both words matter—being free of the small ego self, and doing something useful. Of course not everyone can be "selfless" all the time, and you can't be empty of ego every moment of every day, but you can use breath and meditation to be as empty as possible. A daily practice prepares you to touch that compassionate emptiness very quickly.

Meditation and awareness of the breath will let you help others from a place of emptiness. It is important to be empty because pain adheres to pain. If you bring your own pain with you, the pain of others can cling to you, leaving you overwhelmed or burned out. But why did you bring your own pain? The person suffering doesn't need your tears. She needs your joy and your emptiness.

A great saint, Ramana Maharshi, talked about putting a pitcher full of pure water on a shelf. Everyone comes with a ladle and drinks, and eventually the pitcher will dry out and crack. But if you immerse that pitcher in the waters of the Mother, anyone can come and take as much as they want. You'll constantly be giving, but you'll always be full. If you nourish yourself, you can keep giving and giving. You can learn to drink while you pour. You'll understand how closely prosperity and generosity are entwined.

As you give, commit yourself to serve everyone as best you can and judge no one.

When you go to serve, it is absolutely not about you. And yet, it is not *not* about you. It is about love. Love does not have a certain amount of time or space. It just is.

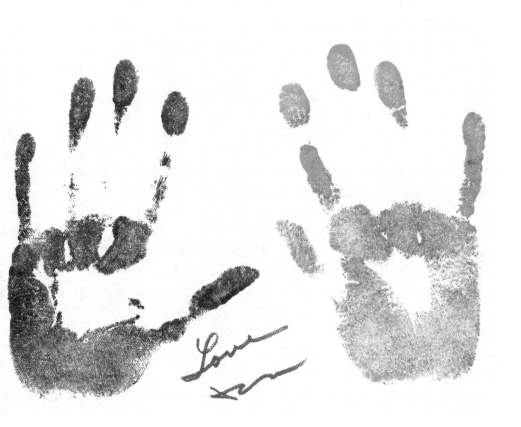

Ma Jaya's Hands

The Healing Breath of Noticing *Healing begins with noticing—noticing your own pain or the pain of others, noticing emotional pain as well as physical pain.*

As you practice this breath, you are practicing the art of inner listening, inner seeing, and inner feeling. This breath allows you to hear the song in yourself that allows you to live with greater compassion for yourself and others.

In the body there are pathways of energy. After some practice with the breath, blockages to these channels will begin to melt away and healing can occur.

Healing is always in the moment. Begin by aligning yourself, becoming comfortable in your body.

The Healing Breath of Noticing

Sit comfortably, keeping your back straight without being rigid. Close your eyes.

Begin to follow and connect with your breath. Let your mind relax.

Begin to notice tensions that arise. Become aware of pain or distractions, notice sounds and thoughts, and allow them to come and go like waves on the ocean.

Place the palm of your hand on your belly and feel the natural rhythm of your breath.

As you center yourself in your breathing, notice what sensations take you away from the breath. Keep returning to the breath.

This is the beginning of healing. You are allowing the body to show you how to open.

Explore the body, scan the body, and feel the areas that ask for healing. Keep bringing the breath to that area. Just by noticing, you are releasing tension and allowing healing to happen.

When you are finished, return your attention to your heart space. Let your heart open as it will. Come out of meditation quietly and kindly.

Healing Hands *With practice you will learn how to bring healing power to others. You do not own this healing power; it is the power of the Mother flowing through you. You are training your own hands to be the healing hands of the Mother.*

If you touch someone with the intention to heal, remember to invoke the Mother as you do, and thank her when you finish. End by rinsing your hands in cold water to release any negativity.

Healing Hands

Place your hands in your lap, palms up. Begin to breathe slowly in and out of your spiritual heart. Focus on the in-breath.

Relax on the out-breath, and let the Mother accept your breath.

With increasing awareness of your hands, take a breath in, visualizing the shakti flowing into your palms, warming them. Feel the same warmth in your spiritual heart.

Feel shakti flowing out of your palms and into the universe.

Begin to breathe in and out the top of your head.

Continue this sequence for several minutes. Keep directing the breath from your heart to your hands, and then out the top of your head.

When you are done, rub your palms together quickly. Their heat will release the healing power. Place your hands on your own body where you need healing; or, with your hands in your lap, palms up, send the healing of your heart to anyone.

If you come into this awareness before you touch others, you will be able to feel that flow continue as you work.

Aging Beautifully *Often a human being is off balance. This is because there are certain times of the day when you breathe more through one nostril or the other.*

When you can be awake enough to balance the breath through both nostrils, then you can be quiet enough to feel your essential self in every moment of your life.

You can also slow the aging process. You begin aging beautifully. Instead of being off balance, you will be in balance with the universal song and the universal rhythm.

Aging Beautifully

Begin by trying to feel in which nostril the breath is stronger, and even it out. As you do the following practice, keep this awareness.

Breathe in for the count of 5, aware that you are breathing in the Mother's prana.

Hold the breath for the count of 7, repeating the name of your Beloved as you count.

Let the breath out for the count of 5.

Keep the breath out for the count of 5, and start again.

Repeat this cycle at least seven times.

Feel the release of tiredness on the out-breath and welcome newness with the in-breath.

When you finish, check again; if your breath is still out of balance, gently align it again. Come into balance.

Avoiding Burn-Out: The Chidakash

Pain adheres to pain, and so if you bring your own pain into a sick person's room, their pain can stick to yours and weigh you down. Caregivers are familiar with this as "burn-out." They chose to enter a helping profession, but after seeing too much pain they may develop a crust around the heart to protect themselves. Those who take care of a sick family member or friend may have a similar experience. No matter how great the love, it's hard to remain open week after week, year after year.

How do you stay open, how do you give love again and again, and yet not be crushed by the pain of others? The answer came from Swami Nityananda of Ganeshpuri, who taught the lessons of the "chidakash,"[6] or "sky of consciousness."

The fourth chakra, the heart, is all about love, but it is often an emotional love. Swami taught that there is another heart space just above the head, a space of cool, unattached love. When you feel overwhelmed by the pain of others, you can focus here and continue to serve. Detachment does not mean not caring. It is quite the opposite. It means caring enough not to react, caring enough not to bring your own pain with you, caring enough to do whatever needs to be done. You will know that whatever situation you face, it is not about you, it is about those you seek to help. With practice, you can enter this space very quickly, staying calm and focused, even in a crisis.

---

6   This is sometimes spelled *"hrid akasha."*

Avoiding Burn-Out: The Chidakash

Breathe into the heart space in the center of your chest, in and out until you feel a spreading warmth. This is the warmth of your heart, awakened by your desire to help.

Now escort your breath to the top of your head, and breathe out into the space of chidakash, the heart space just above the head.

Repeat three times, breathing into the spiritual heart and out the top of the head. Then stay in that space over the head.

You have entered a cool space of detachment. Keep the breath and your awareness over the head while you deal with another person's pain of any kind.

When you are alone at the end of the day, come back to your earthly heart and breathe in and out deeply, relaxing into yourself.

Let yourself feel any emotion from the day. If tears come, allow them.

BETWEEN BREATHS

No Separation

The Mother speaks not to your mind, but to your heart.

All day and all night the Mother speaks to you.

Yet she never speaks as loud as she does when you serve others. Give all you have, and the Mother will fill you again and again.

When you serve one person, you serve all peoples of the world. When you pray for another to be healed, you are also healing yourself.

When you practice acceptance of all people and always love unconditionally, then you understand that everyone is part of the whole. The universal whole cannot exist without every part of it — and we are all part of it.

Everything is interrelated.

Nothing is too small or too big.

There is no division of life.

CHAPTER SEVEN

Mindfulness and the Moment

Negativity cannot live in the moment.

Each breath comes in one time and goes out one time. The sun comes up each day and disappears each night. If you watch the sun come up and give thanks for your life, you could change your perspective and change the way you act. If you watch your breath coming in and out, you can feel how life runs through you.

Wherever you are, this moment is the only chance you have to appreciate this moment. The moment is truly miraculous. Yet, sadly, it can be ignored or overlooked. Awareness of the breath is the way to begin to live in the moment.

We can train ourselves to be mindful of the present moment. That means being aware of what is happening right now, noticing the flow of life as it is happening. When you are mindful, your whole day becomes a dance. There is only the moment, far beyond shadows of thoughts.

When you sit in meditation, let yourself connect with the breath of now. As thoughts arise, label them and let them go. Remind yourself, "It is just a thought." Thoughts have no roots; they cannot hurt you unless you let them.

You are not your thoughts, you are not your past, you are not your future; you are the moment that you breathe in and out now. Stop for a moment, look around you, and feel the texture of this moment. Most of the time, our negativity is linked to past pain or future fears. It is not in the now.

So where do habitual negative thoughts come from? For the most part they are projections of the ego, which keeps you away from your higher self. When you believe in the ego's thoughts, ego becomes your master.

Thoughts constantly arise. Don't try to stop them, just begin to accentuate the positive thoughts by thinking them by choice. Now they become *your* thoughts, not ego's thoughts or karma's thoughts. By mastering the art of deliberate thought, you can loosen the hold of your small ego. As you breathe in, let the positive thoughts take center stage. As you breathe out, let all thoughts go, both positive and negative. When the negative tries to overcome you, do not argue with yourself. Just keep breathing in and out accentuating the positive thought.

If your mind is running wild, learn to firmly say "STOP." Take a breath, and move forward in a quieter space. You can also say, "Not now." Or you can play with the thoughts as if they were circus acts, and like the master of ceremonies ask, "Next…?" Or, you can confuse the mind by asking yourself, "I wonder what my next thought will be?" Or you can use the mind against itself, for example by counting backwards from one thousand. And finally, you can use the breath to flood your mind with love, and watch the small thoughts drown.

There are many techniques. One or another may work best for you, but they all *do* work. And all of a sudden, you are just here. It truly is simple, just coming back to the life you have.

Don't slip off into never-never land. There's no such thing as a psychic place where you will feel God in a different way other than what's right in front of you. It's a mystical journey, but it's also a very sensible journey, this journey of awareness.

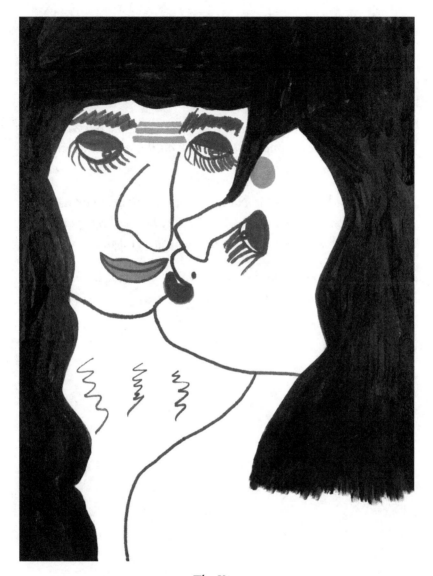

The Kiss

Be Still *In yoga classes you may hear, "Watch your breath." What does this really mean? It is more like* feel *your breath.*

You can consciously breathe into your heart, or you can start by focusing on the subtle touch of the breath on the space between the upper lip and the nostrils.

If you can hold this focus, it will take you into subtle awareness. If you can't keep that awareness, or if the path ever begins to feel too dry or abstract, then come back to your heart again.

It doesn't matter how you find the stillness—just find it. This breath will lead you deeper into meditation.

Be Still

Just begin to watch your breath. As you find yourself becoming calm, begin to count. Do not worry if you lose your place, just start again.

Say to yourself:

Breathing in, one

Breathing out, one

Breathing in, two

Breathing out, two....

Do this until the tenth breath, and then start again.

After several rounds of this, bring your awareness to a focus in the center of your heart. Begin to breathe in and out of the heart deeply and fully, but keep up the counting practice.

As you keep up this counting practice, other thoughts will begin to drop away. Behind the counting is just stillness. After a while, even the counting will begin to drown in the stillness.

Then be still, and let the breath do what it may.

If you are doing this at night before sleep, then just lie down and feel the Mother's silent embrace.

Subtle Awareness *Pranayama often includes alternate nostril breathing, using the hands to close off one side of your nose while breathing through the other.[7] It is also possible to develop enough focus that you can actually direct the breath through the nostrils without using your hands.*

Breathing this way takes a lot of concentration, as you learn subtle awareness. With enough practice, your ability to focus will eventually touch every part of your life. You will bring balance to your brain and energy to your body.

---

7   This practice is known as *anuloma viloma*.

Subtle Awareness

Without touching the nostrils with the hands, direct the breath into the right nostril, then direct it to the third eye point at the center of your forehead. Pause there briefly, and breathe back out the right nostril.

And do the same thing starting on the left: Breathe into the left nostril, pause in the third eye, and breathe out the left.

Repeat, alternating nostrils.

If you can, do this for five minutes. If you can't, then even a couple of rounds of this breath will help you feel calmness surround you.

Simplicity *Pure mindfulness meditation, just watching the breath, will eventually bring you to a space of compassion, but combining it with a heart breath opens the heart more quickly. This breath combines the simple practice of mindfulness with a heart-opening breath.*

It also helps you release staleness of any kind, especially karmic staleness. Karma is always stale, since it comes from past actions. Mindfulness brings you to the present moment, where karma does not rule you.

If you do this early in the day, you can watch how complications arise all day long. As they do, return again and again to the simplicity of the breath.

Simplicity

Start to pay attention to the exhalation, without controlling or measuring the breath.

When you can do that, breathe out more deeply, contracting the belly muscles, releasing all the staleness in your life out into the universe.

When you are comfortable with contracting the belly muscles on every out-breath, begin to do it harder. Not too hard! Be gentle with yourself.

By breaking the habitual pattern of your breath, you are also breaking the patterns that have been created by yesterday's thoughts and tomorrow's worries.

Stay aware while you allow the breath to return to its own rhythm.

Do not worry if you get a little light-headed. You are just learning how to focus. There's no need to be afraid, because you always have the breath to come back to.

The Mindful Heart

This breath quiets the mind and frees you. Let the essence of the breath, moment by moment, merge into the open field of awareness. Merge with all that you are, embrace all of yourself, and make room for the moment exactly as it is. Thoughts come and go, sounds come and go, doubts come and go. Let them; these things will dissolve as you continue to watch your breath.

While some practices lead you to chakras above your head, mindfulness consists of being fully present in this body, this moment. And so this breath does not lead you to the crown chakra or beyond.

With practice, this simple breath can become a big part of your life.

The Mindful Heart

Sitting straight, breathe into the center of your chest, filling the chest cavity with a fearless breath. Hold the breath gently, allowing yourself to open.

Breathe out slowly, very slowly, focusing on the out-breath.

Again, breathe in deeply, holding the breath without strain.

Breathing out, the mind may wander, but do not judge yourself.

Dive deeper, continuing to breathe in and out of the chest cavity. Do five breaths with this focus.

Then breathe into the throat chakra for five breaths. Breathing in, know you are breathing in; breathing out, know you are breathing out.

Breathe in and out of the third eye for five breaths.

Now guide yourself to the base of the spine for five breaths.

Take five breaths in and out of the second chakra.

Allow the breath to rise. Continue to take five breaths in and out of each chakra ending at the forehead. Each chakra may bring its own thoughts and feelings. Be aware of them, and let them pass.

Then repeat this entire cycle five times.

Then sit in your own beauty, becoming more and more aware of all that surrounds you and all that is within you.

Silence *Silence is much more than the absence of sound.*

There are levels and levels of silence.

Your soul calls for silence so you can hear it.

Your soul calls for stillness so you can feel it.

Your soul calls for your attention so you can be it.

The soul never dies. It just always was, is, and will be.

Silence

Sit in the stillness and become aware of your thoughts passing through. Watch your thoughts as a silent witness.

You are not your thoughts.

Find a space between a thought passing away and a thought appearing. Look for that tiny time between thoughts, and prolong it. Do not try too hard. It will come to you with practice.

Do this for about five minutes and then watch your breath, without trying to control it. Become more aware of the spaces *between* your thoughts.

Bring your awareness to your spiritual heart and think of your whole heart chakra as a wide-open space.

Rest in the spaces between the breaths and between the thoughts.

Just lose yourself in this space of silent meditation.

BETWEEN BREATHS

The Moment

When you judge yourself or others, you stop yourself from melting into the oneness of the universe. The mind concentrates on the things it understands and therefore stops the flow.

This is the way of the ego—to always keep the mind going and going and making new stories to stop you from merging with the oneness.

The past takes on a life of its own, which keeps changing as your story changes.

Time creates history. Meditation creates the moment.

CHAPTER EIGHT

Letting Go

*The breath can bring you to the original truth of
who you are.*

Spiritual life is all about letting go. You learn to let go of that
which is impermanent because impermanence equals *samsara*,
or illusion. Samsara is, for instance, the body. Every hour our
bones are changing, our skin changes, our cells change, and
eventually we die.

When you attach yourself to objects that change, you cannot
understand the beauty and value of the changeless soul.

Your soul is already perfect; your task is to let go of anything
and everything that clouds that perfection. An earlier chapter
was about letting go of stress and tension, but there is more to
give up—staleness, negativity, anger, jealousy, procrastination,
attachment, and so much more.

You may have tried to give up these things, but they arise again.
The breath can help you break old, deep patterns that follow
you from situation to situation, and even from life to life. In
giving up samskaras, you are actually loosening the karmic
bonds that keep you cycling from one negative space to another,
around and around, perhaps for lifetimes.

You may feel as if you are not in charge of your own life, and
perhaps you're not if you are just running along in the deep
ruts made by karma. Most of the time, we don't choose, we just

react. That's karma—cause and effect, cause and effect, cause and effect, again and again.

One important way to freedom is to learn non-reaction. You can train yourself to hesitate just a split second between action and reaction, or between stimulus and response. That moment of hesitation is where your freedom lies. It is actually a gap in the laws of karma, because you are choosing how to respond.

There are many angers, many jealousies, and many things to cling to, but every time you give up a tiny piece of a karmic pattern, you take another step on the path of freedom.

Meditation is one key, because for a little while you commit to reacting to nothing—not your thoughts, your boredom, your emotions, your back pain, not any of it.

Breath is the other key, because the more you breathe in the prana of the universe, the more you breathe out what you do not need. Karma lives in the body as staleness, meaning old thoughts, old emotions, old reactions, old pain. When we release staleness, we are freeing ourselves from karmic bonds.

The out-breath is important because how well we live our lives is not so much about what we take in — it's more about what we let go, let go, let go, and what we don't take back. Each moment can be an experience of holding on to pain, fear, anger, and negativity of all kinds. Or you can live so that each moment is a letting go of anything you don't need.

You can intentionally offer anything up to the Mother in her form of Kali, or you can just let it go into the universe, where the Mother takes it. Whether or not Kali or the Black Mother is mentioned in the practices that follow, just know that she is always there and always ready to help you give up anything you don't need.

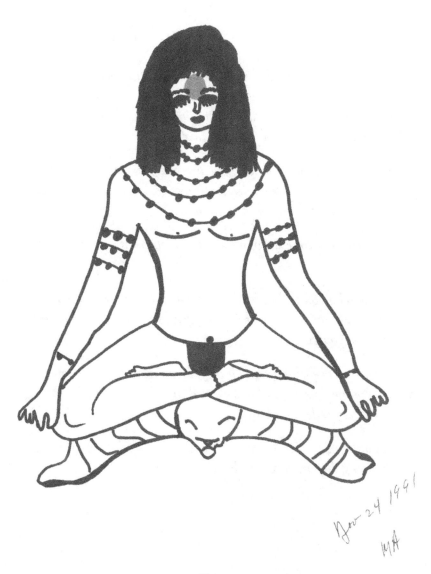

Shiva

Forgiveness *An ancient teaching from the time of the Buddha is, "Hatred never ceases by hatred, but by love alone is healed. This is an ancient and eternal law." Forgiveness allows us to release the past and go on with our lives.*

Forgiveness is a process, a very long process. It is work of the heart, but first we have to make a decision to let go. If we can forgive, we do not carry the poison of hate within us.

Forgiveness frees your self of poison and replaces it with self-worth and joy.

Becoming who you truly are affects the world more than anything else you could do. As you ask for forgiveness from others, you must also forgive yourself.

The next practice leads you to a very deep meditation. As you strip yourself of the poison you have carried around with you for so long, you can feel freedom and joy.

A deep hurt may have many layers. Allow yourself time to let go, gently doing this practice a little bit each day.

Forgiveness

Sitting in a comfortable position with the back straight and relaxed, let the eyes close gently and bring your attention to your breath. Deeply breathe in and out of the area around your chest, letting the breath be centered in the space of the heart.

Breathe in for the count of 9.

Hold the breath in for the count of 9.

Breathe out for the count of 9.

Hold the breath out for the count of 9.

Keep repeating this pattern. All the while, ask the universal Mother for forgiveness for hurting anyone or for hurting yourself. Remember the sorrows you have caused yourself, and let them go on the wings of the breath. Over and over say to yourself, "I forgive myself, I forgive myself."

Keep breathing with awareness, breathing into your chest and feeling the beauty of forgiveness. Feel the heart softening with the awareness of the breath.

Then just sit quietly with the intention of forgiveness. Ask of the universe, "May I be filled with love and acceptance." Then let the thoughts come and go, blessing each thought as you are filled with forgiveness for others and yourself.

Keep breathing with awareness as you live your life with compassion for all things and for yourself.

The Jasmine Breath *Anxiety is rooted in lack of self-worth. Every time you begin to dwell on your shortcomings, you can choose instead to breathe in the warmth of the Mother and the scent of love. The next practice includes visualization, but you can also put your sense of smell to work.*

Every time you are caught by fears for the future, you can use the breath to bring you back to the now. Let go of both past and future.

The Jasmine Breath

Sitting quietly with your eyes closed, visualize yourself in the middle of a large bed of white, sweet-smelling jasmine flowers.

Feel the warmth of the sun reflecting off the flowers and embracing you. Slowly draw up the warmth into your body. Soak it up the way a sponge soaks up water. Smell the jasmine.

Breathe in and out as you bathe in the light of the sun. Relax your neck, back, and shoulders. Feel your whole body shed tension. Your physical and spiritual being begins to be at peace.

Breathe in for a count of 8.

Breathe out for a count of 6.

Then breathe in and out of the heart three times without counting the seconds, absorbing the light inside of your heart.

Relax and breathe naturally.

Repeat this sequence three times.

Sit quietly, continuing to feel the sun and smell the jasmine.

Giving Up Fears *Phobias are like roots, and some are so
deeply embedded that they are actually samskaras, deep patterns
that may continue from lifetime to lifetime. They can have real and
debilitating effects on our lives, yet many of us hang on to them
tightly. Sometimes we forget what we are afraid of and we go right
to a space of repressed anxiety.*

*To bring your fears out into the open, begin to name them,
speaking them aloud. Or write them, if you prefer. The door to the
unconscious flies open; words and fears come out and are caught in
the net of the moment.*

*After you recognize some of your fears, you can use the breath to
release them. Some breaths, like this one, are very simple; you don't
have to hold your breath or count. But when you add the power of
the breath to any kind of self-inquiry, it becomes easier to let go of
what you don't need.*

Giving Up Fears

Sit comfortably with your back straight and your eyes closed. Take five deep breaths as you begin to relax into a meditative state.

Now ask yourself, truly ask yourself, "What is the cause of my fear?" Let the answers come from deep within, not from the ego mind. Then fix your focus on a light so bright within your heart that the brightness warms your whole being.

Nothing can exist in our lives without us giving it energy. When energy stagnates, we can begin to release it with the out-breath. Breathe out your fears, and let them dissolve into light.

Does this seem too simple? Sometimes the simplest path is the best, and it is the ego that craves complication.

Desire to Be Right
Do people listen to you when you speak? If they don't, do you feel deeply hurt? How much energy or shakti are you giving to this particular kind of hurt?

If this is a pattern for you, it's a sign that you may have gotten caught in the desire to be right.

The desire to be right is a karmic space, a seemingly safe place to retreat and hide from the world. It seems safe because it is familiar, but in fact it is a trap.

The desire to be right can cause you to not listen to others, and at times to not even listen to your own intuition.

The desire to be right can destroy relationships or start wars.

It is a very lonely space, walled in by your own self-righteous thoughts.

Even if you are right, is it worth it? Most of the time, the only person you hurt with this habit is yourself.

This practice uses the power of the breath combined with self-examination to let go of righteousness and replace it with love.

Desire to Be Right

Think of someone you are disagreeing with, or someone who seems never to listen to you. The first one who comes to mind is usually the best one to work with. Visualize this person, and possibly imagine a short conversation.

Meanwhile, breathe deeper and deeper, but slowly and relaxed. Resist the temptation to give in to the tight, angry breath of anger.

Take a little vacation from this karmic space.

You are learning to focus on the thoughts you choose to have, not the ones presented to you by your lower mind.

Now begin to focus on the in-breath and use it to wrap the other person and yourself in love.

When the negative tries to overcome you, do not argue with yourself, just keep breathing in and out, accentuating the positive.

When you're ready, switch your attention more to the out-breath. Let all thoughts go as you breathe out. The walls you have built begin to crumble.

Continue to use this practice as you gradually give up the habitual desire to be right.

BETWEEN BREATHS

The Black Mother Kali

In seeking freedom through breath and meditation, always remember the Mother Kali. She devours pain, devours truth, devours falseness, devours all that is, and just leaves the purity of the heart.

She wanders the skies in search of any kind of sorrow so she can absorb it inside of herself.

You don't even have to know her name, but you must believe that there is a Mother and that this Mother will wrap her arms around you and hold you no matter what. She will love you and touch you and give you compassion, and in the same breath she will strip the flesh away from your bones and leave you free.

She does this because nothing, no pain in your life, no guilt, no desire, no attachment, is so big that it is worth forgetting God.

Why is Kali dark and terrifying? That is *your* darkness, which she takes from you. She takes from you what you do not need. As she grows darker, you grow lighter. In her blackness, which is darker than any darkness in you, the Black Mother consumes what you don't need on your journey—if you offer it to her.

CHAPTER NINE

Practical Breaths

It takes a lot of courage to be happy.

The breath is a practical tool for changing your life. You already have abundant experience of this. First, your mother and your kindergarten teacher may have told you to take a deep breath and count to ten when you were on the brink of an angry outburst. Later in life, you may have learned about aligning body and breath in a yoga class, or singing, or sports. Some people have discovered the breath as a way to work with physical pain, for example in natural childbirth. For some, breath is linked with positive affirmations as part of a healing process. Others have discovered that the power of the breath can be linked to the power of prayer. The point is, it doesn't matter very much what your original goal was, or why you first become aware of the breath and its power to change your life. It still works!

Pranayama is about learning to direct prana, your life force, in whatever direction you choose. This chapter offers some specific breaths that can help you work with specific problems like addiction, obesity, and procrastination.

Much pain arises from habitual patterns. Some of your patterns feel so deep that they seem to have been with you since childhood, or even to be determined by your karma from another life. No matter the source, changing your breath can change your habits and your patterns.

Try these breaths for whatever you want to accomplish, and at the same time be prepared for deeper changes. Yes, deeper changes can happen. Breath and meditation bring you to the full openness of the moment, the now. Meditation is not about making something happen; meditation is about being there in the moment and being aware.

Just because you're on a spiritual path, it shouldn't stop you from using every tool to make your ordinary life better. You certainly did not enter spiritual life to be sad! Spiritual practice should never be tedious or boring.

What does happiness mean to you? Happiness could be losing ten pounds, or improving a relationship, or finally finishing that project. Or, you might define happiness as discovering your eternal soul, giving up all attachments, and merging into the joy of the universe. Using any of the tools for transformation that are available to us, we can actually do *all* these things, whether we think of them as "worldly" or "spiritual."

It's not really either/or, worldly happiness vs. spiritual happiness, so don't pass judgment on your own hopes. And don't forget to give thanks. As you lie down to sleep tonight, think of the many blessings you have received this day. Gratitude keeps you open to receive the next gift. When you do not have gratitude, you stop the process of receiving.

As you try these breaths, remember that the Mother holds you tight to her breast as you breathe in the newness of joy inside of your heart and the heart of the world.

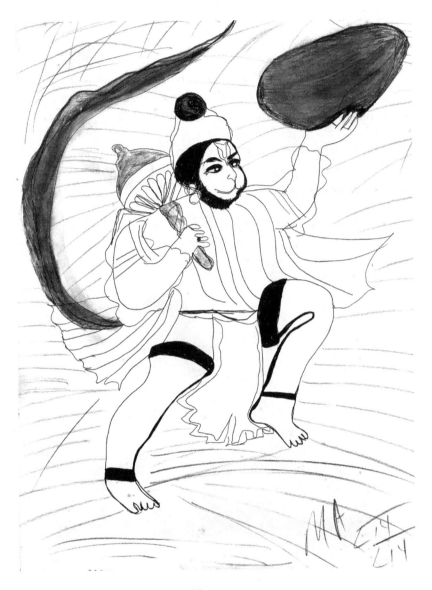

Hanuman

Prayer and Blessing *You can learn to breathe in light and breathe out a blessing. Breathing in with awareness, you are nourishing yourself. Breathing out, you are nourishing others.*

The next practice gives you a tool to bless the world, perhaps combining it with a prayer for peace. You can also use it to send love to someone in need.

Prayer is love, and love is prayer.

Prayer and Blessing

As you think of a person you want to pray for, breathe light in and out, going deeper and deeper each time.

Take your time and actually feel this light. It is the light of the Mother, which can eat any darkness.

Say over and over, "I am breathing in the great light of the Mother." She will take your breath and filter out what you do not need.

As you breathe out, say to yourself, "I am bringing love to the world." Or you could name a specific person or situation.

Keep doing this breathing until you feel at peace with yourself.

Feel the wonderment of love as the breath goes out on its own and touches the earth.

Breath to Lose Weight *This is a variant on the* sitali *breath, a cooling breath that is part of many yoga practices. The key is to curl the tongue into a shape like a trough, a tube, and stick it out of your mouth a little bit, so that when you breathe in it feels like you're drinking through a straw. (The tongue needs to be curled only on the inhalation.)*

Not everyone can curl the tongue like this. If you can't, visualize the curved shape, close your lips part way, and feel the breath in the back of your throat.

Breath to Lose Weight

Sit comfortably, with a straight back. Curl your tongue into a tube. Take a slow, deep breath in and visualize that the breath is all going into your head, as if your head is filling up like a balloon.

Relax your tongue and close your mouth. Hold the breath as long as it's comfortable, then slowly breathe out. Visualize the breath leaving through the top of your head.

Breathing in through your curled tongue, fill your belly with breath until you feel like you just ate a very big meal. Relax your tongue. Hold the breath as long as you're comfortable, and then breathe out the top of your head.

And keep going, alternating one breath in your head and one breath in your belly.

Just remember to always curl the tongue as you breathe in, and always breathe out the top of your head.

Conquering Addictions   *If you are filled with prana, what more do you need?*

With that in mind, try using this practice to help you out of any addiction.

It takes time to end addictions, so be patient. It is said that it takes forty days to break a habit, but of course not everyone is the same. Still, with that in mind, you can set the intention to do this every day for forty days.

Conquering Addictions

Begin with a triple in-breath, through the nose, three quick in-breaths without breathing out.

Hold the breath in your belly or third chakra as long as comfortable.

Breathe out strongly but slowly, using your stomach muscles to squeeze out any staleness.

Do this cycle three times, but not more than that.

Ending Procrastination

Procrastination, or unfulfilled intent, can ruin your life. You have so many good ideas, so many loving impulses, and you kill them by always saying "I'll do it later...." Tomorrow turns into "next week, next year..." until you realize you have grown old and you have missed out on the richness of life.

If you believe in reincarnation, you may even catch yourself thinking, "I can do it next life," and indeed that's how karma works. What you don't do this life will be waiting for you in another form, but it won't be any easier next time.

Do this breath for forty days, and watch procrastination dissolve.

Ending Procrastination

Slowly count backwards from 29. Do this three times,
feeling the breath become very subtle. You almost feel the
breath stopping.

If you lose your place, try a few more times and then go on. You
will get it after some practice.

When you are finished counting, repeat the next cycle five times:

Breathe in this subtle breath to the count of 7.

Hold it for 7.

Breathe out for the count of 7.

Hold out for the count of 7.

When you finish, breathe in and out of your spiritual heart for
a few minutes. If the breath remains very subtle, you may need
to take a few deep in-breaths to get yourself ready to go on with
your day.

BETWEEN BREATHS

Miracles

Miracles begin to happen when you are free with an open heart. Shakti, the force of the Mother, is in all things, and there is never a lack of anything when you know how to open to the universe's abundance.

Feel the warmth of receiving and the beauty of giving.

Concentrate on the receiving, even the receiving of being healed by the universe. Allow this to happen to you.

Go beyond your limitations and open to the joy that the Mother wants for you.

You have the ability to transform yourself into a being of light. You are the miracle that you seek.

CHAPTER TEN

Ego, Awareness, Intuition

The ego's self-importance is erased by the breath.

At every step on the spiritual path, you have an ego that will fight you. It will tell you that you are too tired or too busy to do your yoga or your meditation or your breath work. It will tell you that you are worthless, and then it will turn around and tell you that you are the greatest. It will take love and turn it into attachment. It will take everything good in your life and fill you with doubt.

The ego gives birth to a limited mind; when you give attention to the limited mind, you lead a very limited life. It is the ego that stops you from knowing all of your possibilities. It is the ego that comes between you and the heart.

And yet, our true inner voice is always a breath away. We are all born with a spiritual potential of intuitive awareness. The breath will bring you a new awareness of your own hidden consciousness. Anything that you need to know from the universe is deep in your heart, and in meditation you begin to realize how much of this hidden potential you can uncover and use. With patience, you can feel the lotus opening.

There are many dimensions within you that are waiting to unfold like the lotus. These dimensions permeate reality. You may not be aware of them, yet your intuitive mind knows they are there. As you learn to escort your wandering thoughts back to your breath, you will go deeper and deeper.

The more you can diminish the ego's hold on you, the closer you can come to your higher self. The breath allows you to grow toward it as you go deeper and deeper inside of yourself.

Do not give up on yourself. Your intuition is awakening. As your breath brings you deeper and deeper within your own being, you will start to trust yourself more and more. But when the ego is strong, how little of the universe you allow into your life!

Your ego stands between you and the whole universal experience of the heart.

Your ego stands between you and the glorious experience of love and all the dimensions that love brings you.

Awareness lies in your heart, waiting for you to find it and use it.

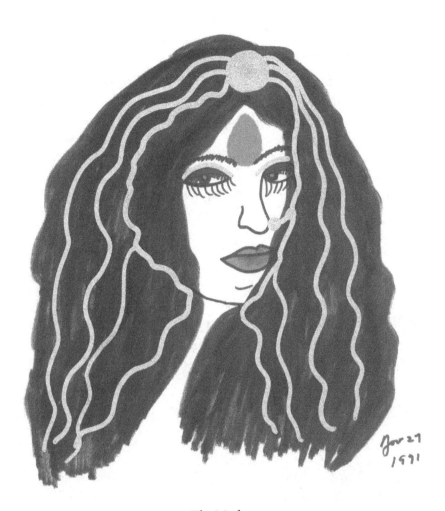

The Mother

Awareness *You can grow strong and sure if you concentrate in the sixth chakra during meditation. Here is a simple practice to help you trust your spiritual intuition.*

However, this is not about opening yourself to psychic visions or developing magical powers, both of which we usually associate with the "third eye." It is possible to get stuck in the psychic realms, which can be a distraction on the spiritual path.

Opening the third eye is about learning to trust your spiritual intuition.

It is also about becoming more and more aware of the divinity in all things. Yogi Bhajan would say, "If you can't see God in all, you can't see God at all." That's the understanding the sixth chakra can bring.

Awareness

Using the breath to keep your focus, feel warm light coming in through your forehead. Breathe it in, as if the light was all around you and you could drink it through the third eye.

Look inside yourself and let the light spread through your body. Let it fill you.

On every in-breath, feel light whirling around inside your body.

On every out-breath, send light out through the third eye. There is no darkness, just more light to breathe in.

Do this for about ten minutes. Then let yourself go, and let the breath take care of itself.

As you go into a silent meditation, the light will remain.

What Is My Purpose? *You can clear your mind until there is just you and the Mother. Then your intuition can flow, and in that simple knowing you will find answers to your deepest questions.*

This specific practice offers a way to discover your purpose in life, and you can also adapt it to work with other big questions. You may think you have a million questions; this breath offers a gradual deepening of intuition, not a million quick answers.

Take time to explore deeply. You may find, as you answer one question, that some others no longer need to be asked.

What Is My Purpose?

Start by breathing in and out every chakra, starting at the base of the spine, saying to yourself, "breathing in the first chakra, breathing out the first chakra," and so on. By telling yourself the number of each chakra, you are practicing awareness.

Do this cycle three times.

Sit quietly and let the two worlds come together, the inner world and the outer world.

After a few minutes begin to breathe in and out of the heart chakra. Do this for eleven breaths.

Then sit quietly, focusing on your heart. Feel the knowing enter your spiritual heart in the middle of your chest.

With great awareness ask, "What is my purpose in life?"

Sit quietly for up to fifteen minutes and listen deeply, still asking your question.

Do this for three days straight, and do not worry if you do not get an answer right away. If there is still no answer, then let it go for three days, and then do the meditation again for three days. Keep meditating on the question, and an answer will come.

Soon you will find a new intuitive knowing has entered into you.

Trust Your Intuition *Each of us has male and female energies within us. Trusting ourselves opens all the channels to both energies.*

Whether you are man or woman, it is the female energy that develops trust and intuition. The ego keeps you off balance by leading you to avoid either your male or female aspect. With awareness, both aspects meet in the center of the heart. Living in a state of consciousness of love keeps you balanced no matter what life throws at you.

Trust Your Intuition

Take a deep breath and then exhale slowly, letting yourself relax.

Do this for eleven breaths.

When you relax, you become at home with your two energies, male and female.

Keep breathing deeply and notice how your breath is filled with a loving energy, and see how it circulates to every cell of your body. Begin to realize that you have access to this energy any time you want.

Open yourself with each in-breath. Allow yourself to absorb it. Be absorbed in it. Feel positive and confident with every in-breath.

Now pay attention to your out-breath, only your out-breath. Feel all tension leave your body. Feel all darkness disappear out of your body. Any negative thoughts that you ever have experienced can leave on the out-breath.

Now as each breath comes in, say to yourself "In." As each breath flows out, say "Out."

Do this for as long as you are comfortable.

Then take a deep breath and notice how much more relaxed you are, how much more balanced you are.

You have just awakened both your male and female energy. Now you are ready to live in the moment.

The Sky Mind of the Chidakash *The chapter on healing included a breath to help caregivers avoid burn-out by entering the chidakash, a space of compassionate detachment. There is actually more to it than that.*

Chidakash means "sky of consciousness" or "sky-mind." It is the clear mind of pure consciousness—very precise, very clear, never changing. Sky-mind is the brightness of the sun, but it is usually covered by clouds.

Like the soul, the sky-mind is unchanged by joy or sorrow, sickness or health; it is beyond emotion, beyond attachment, beyond reaction.

All emotion, even joy, keeps you spreading yourself along the ground of your life, and you may forget about the sky. Meanwhile the ego cries out, "Dwell here, don't look up, for here you will be much more comfortable." And, yes, you certainly will be, because we are all used to being in our patterns of emotion.

You can give up attachment, you can let go of emotion, and you can stop reacting to every passing cloud. You can learn to live in the chidakash.

But isn't love an emotion?

There is emotional love that we feel in the spiritual heart, and there is the chidakash, a higher love that is free of attachment. Once you know both spaces, you will be able to move between them.

The Sky Mind of the Chidakash

Picture the sky-mind, the chidakash, above your head. This is the realm the Mother Kundalini reaches toward. The breath opens her path.

Starting at the base of the spine, breathe deeply into each chakra, feeling that you are stretching and reaching toward the freedom of the soul.

Breath in to the base of the spine and out the second chakra. Breathe in to the second chakra and out the third, and continue.

When you reach the center of your chest, hold your breath in the heart, feeling a warmth spread. Take your time, and then breathe out through the throat.

When you reach the top of your head, you are leaving the space of attachment. Follow the breath out, and rest there about two inches above the top of your head. You may feel distant, and yet present.

Your breath may become very subtle, and you may feel you are hardly breathing. Even so, keep directing the breath and your awareness as an upward flow.

From the space above your head, look up, visualize the night sky, the stars, and feel the greatness of the universe. Rest here and allow the subtle breath to lead you where it wants to go.

Come out of this meditation slowly, for it is quite powerful. Bring your awareness to the center of your chest and take a few deeper breaths to ground you.

When you are done, bow your head and give thanks for your life.

BETWEEN BREATHS

The Inner Universe

When you focus inside, the inner universe begins to still any hectic movements. Thus the light shines within as time begins to stop. This is internal breathing riding on eternal time. The breath seems to stop, and yet internal breathing goes on and on.

A feeling of lightness comes over you as you commune with the breathless state that is always within.

Space bows out, and outer creation and inner creation come together. Samsara ceases to exist and the vastness of wisdom bursts forth. Your own pure soul wishes to communicate with you through your higher mind. We feel this as intuition.

You all have divine love flowing through you. While the ego continually tells you what to do or not to do, divine love speaks to your heart, and you just *know* what to do.

The Mother's path of love does not follow the ways of the ego.

CHAPTER ELEVEN

Life, Death, Samadhi

You do not have to go on dreaming of liberation.
You already have it within you.

You have heard again and again about the perfection of your own soul, you have heard that the universe is within you, and you have been told that you can overcome every obstacle.

This is all true! But do you *believe* it? Sure, you are "made in the image of God," but meanwhile the baby is crying, the car is broken down, the rent is due, and you have a headache. In the course of a lifetime, most of us get only fleeting experiences of our own divinity. It does not have to be like that! With practice, you can expand these moments until they are part of your normal awareness.

In being aware of the breath, you will also become aware of the place of the non-breath, where the body becomes so still, the mind so engrossed in the divine, that the breath is suspended.

As you rise, the breath becomes more and more subtle until you may even feel it has stopped. And sometimes it actually *has* stopped. Of course as soon as you notice you're not breathing, you will start breathing again. You may have felt the breath stop while doing any of the deeper practices in this book. Your body is preparing for samadhi, the deathless state of perfect awareness. Samadhi is the death of the ego, a totally freeing experience; it is letting go, completely, of all attachments, riding the waves of breath, and being very aware and prepared for that moment of non-breath.

It takes very long practice to rest fully in the non-breath, and yet a beginner may at times reach very deep states, so try not to judge what you feel. Every living person has the ability to enter into a space of samadhi. Trust that the Mother knows what she is doing, and step toward her with as much awareness and love as you can muster.

Every breath has death and rebirth in it. When you sit in the silence of meditation, you gradually get used to the death state, and you train your body and mind to handle it. Then, as you begin to live with this awareness, you open a door, a whole new way of life. In the stillness you begin to know yourself.

Then when death arrives, you know what to do. To be conscious of that last breath is ecstasy. It's an orgasm that lasts until your next rebirth, a trembling that never stops, and that's the true meaning of tantra, an idea that has been much misunderstood and mistranslated. Tantra means "continuation." It is the flow of the in-breath and out-breath, the flowing motion of great rivers and of your own blood, or the flow of life and death and life again. More than anything, it is awareness. To be aware of the breath is to be aware in both life and death.

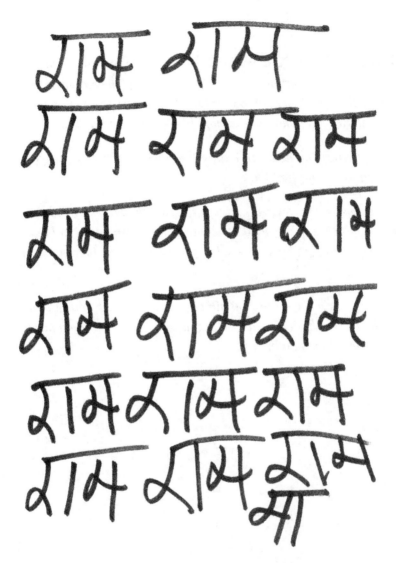

Ma Jaya's Rams

119

Breath and Non-Breath *You may get afraid when you feel your breath getting very subtle or stopping. The ego mind wants you to think you will run out of breath, and it wants you to be so afraid that you don't dare explore higher consciousness.*

This practice will help you realize that there is actually enough breath, and you are OK.

If you ever get too scared and want to stop the process, just breathe out. The mind may tell you to contract and gasp for an in-breath, but breathing out opens everything and restarts the breath easily and naturally.

Here is a practice that seems simple, but it will keep you in touch with the breath all day. It also begins to deepen your awareness of the space of the non-breath.

Breath and Non-Breath

As you read these words, breathe out.

You will have a desire to breathe in; do not.

Breathe out again without breathing in.

Now one more time, breathe out.

Then breathe in deeply.

During the day just breathe out whenever you think of it, and notice how you want to breathe in right away.

Instead, breathe out three or four times on the same out- breath (contracting the belly tightly), and then breathe in deeper than ever before.

See how much you appreciate your in-breath.

Soon you will appreciate every breath you take and those you do not.

Breathing with the Dead

So many perceive death as a finality, but actually death is just an end to a certain form. The breath lives in spirit, and spirit holds the breath for future lives.

Death lives in life and life lives in death. The breath is the interconnection of all things. It is through the breath of the living that the dead live again, even before rebirth.

When you think of someone you have lost, breathe and feel love. Breathe in love and breathe out to the world, again and again. Do not forget to dedicate the breath, and the Mother's ears shall pick up the sound of your dedication and bless you both.

As you open more and more to your breath, you become more and more aware that death has no beginning or ending; you discover that whoever you lost to death is never lost. You are still breathing in their breath. You are still breathing out their breath.

This next breath is not about trying to make contact with the dead in a psychic way. It is about bringing yourself into such a space of light that you can feel for yourself the eternal flow of life and death.

Breathing with the Dead

Breathe in the Mother's breath into the deepest part of your third chakra. Hold the breath and dedicate it to one you have lost, or any one in the world who has left the body.

Then send out from your third eye a great light of yearning to return to the source. During the out-breath feel the great light break up into little sparks, like little perfect diamonds.

Now breathe in deeply such a rich and rare prana that your heart will open wide to receive it. Hold the breath and feel the sparks of the perfect diamonds flow all over your body.

Breathe out and feel the great light break up again, and now breathe in again.

You can start off doing this for five rounds, feeling more and more in touch with those who have left. It is like you are both sharing the banks of great rivers and are drenched in the holy spirit of the sparkling diamonds.

The Original Thought *There is a place inside of you that is one with the breath, and one with every one and every thing. This is the soul, or the original thought. It is the space of simplicity that never changes and always remains.*

You can touch that space any time in your day with this simple practice of awareness.

The Original Thought

Breathe deeply and fully, and breathe out just a little bit longer than you breathed in.

Allow the out-breath to become longer and longer.

Enjoy both breaths, in and out, yet be still, and feel that place between the breaths that never changes.

Breathe, breathe, breathe with awareness. Feel the simplicity of open awareness before thought.

Breathe, breathe, breathe with the greatest amount of love.

The River Breath
As our last breath goes out, according to the laws of nature and the laws of God, something must be breathed in. We breathe out our last breath. Death breathes us in, and holds the breath. So death is a suspension. You have your little breath, which flows continuously in and out, out and in. And there's the bigger breath, life and death, death and life, in one continuous flow. The soul is the breath. Death breathes us in, and the out-breath of death is rebirth. Death's out-breath is the beginning of life.

The River Ganges or Ganga is considered to be the Mother of India, with all of her life-giving bounty. It is auspicious to die near her banks. Dedicate this breath to the river, and feel yourself drenched in a river of life, a river of love, constantly in the flow of being.

She is the destroyer of all impure thoughts. Throw everything in the flowing waters of the Ganga. As life flows into death and death flows into life, the river continues to flow. This is the real meaning of tantra: continuation. No beginning, no ending.

The River Breath is a ratio breath, which means that the counts for in-breath, hold in, out-breath and hold out, are in a specific relationship to each other. We start with a comfortable 2-8-4-2 ratio, but after a little practice you can change to 4-16-8-4.

The River Breath

Close your eyes and feel your heart and the deep silence surrounding you. Especially begin to notice the silence of the out-breath.

Start by breathing in through the nose for a count 2.

Hold the breath while you count to 8.

Slowly contract the belly and release the breath through your mouth while you count to 4.

And hold the breath out while you count to 2.

Repeat.

Start with three cycles and gradually build up, but not more than ten repetitions at one time. You can also increase the count, but keep the ratio. Do not strain or struggle with this breath; it is all about feeling the flow.

After doing the breath, let yourself go into the silence. Get comfortable in silence, and get in the habit of feeling the in-breath flow into the out-breath just as life flows into death and back again.

BETWEEN BREATHS

The River

Children play in my River

Sadhus stay by my River

Temples made of gold by my River

Cows stray all the day by my River

Old men die by my River

Widows cry by my River

1008 candles drift on the leaves that float on my River

They light the hope of many by my River.

River, River, I am thirsty

I am burning, my River

Quench my thirst, my Mother.

I need the River to know her own

Ganga take my children home....

This is the beginning of Ma's long poem "The River," which she started in 1978. She added to it during the rest of her life. A version was published in book form in 1994.

About the Author

Ma Jaya Sati Bhagavati (1940-2012) was a spiritual teacher, mystic, and visionary. She taught that divinity is ultimately beyond words and without form, yet manifests in countless ways to lead us to liberation. All paths of love can lead to spiritual awakening.

Ma Jaya's accomplishments include founding an interfaith community called Kashi Ashram; developing Kali Natha Yoga, a modern system drawn from ancient roots; guiding service projects in India, Uganda, and the US; working to end religious prejudice; supporting the LGBTQ community; overseeing a K-12 school; founding a model community for low-income seniors; and creating a large body of sacred art.

Born into a Jewish family in 1940, Ma Jaya grew up in a cellar apartment in Brighton Beach, Brooklyn, a short walk from the ocean and the famous Coney Island Boardwalk. As a young girl, she found love and solace among the homeless people who lived under the Boardwalk. Welcoming her, they taught her many lessons about life, especially, "There are no throwaway people." She grew up to dedicate her life to humanity.

Enrolling in a weight loss class in 1972 led her to learn a simple yogic breath that would ultimately bring about her spiritual enlightenment. Her personal spiritual journey moved quickly and, at times, chaotically. As a modern urban woman, she tried to live a normal life and raise a family; at the same time, as a person of rare spiritual gifts, she daily opened to a series of mystical visions and experiences. She had experiences first of Jesus Christ, then of Shri Bhagawan Nityananda of Ganeshpuri, and eventually her guru, Shri Neem Karoli Baba. As early as 1973, she began to "teach all ways," as Christ has instructed her to do. She gave a contemporary voice to the great truths that underlie all spiritual paths.

She offered the example of a spiritual life alive with love, faith, creativity, service, and the rituals of many traditions. Emphasizing individual spiritual growth, she taught seekers at all levels and never asked her students to follow any particular set of doctrines or beliefs. Or, as she often said, "This is not a religion!" She encouraged her students to use her teachings within their own faiths or traditions, and to practice kindness.

Ma Jaya began to teach yoga and breath practices in 1973. In 2000 she began to share her yoga teachings more deeply and gave them the name Kali Natha Yoga. Her teachings on karma formed the basis for her book *The 11 Karmic Spaces: Choosing Freedom from the Patterns that Bind You*, which won a gold medal from the Independent Publishers' Association.

In 1976, Ma Jaya moved to Florida and founded Kashi Ashram, a spiritual community that embraces all religious and spiritual paths, where her students continue to teach and serve in her name.

Glossary

Ajna: The sixth chakra, located in the forehead.

Anahata: The fourth chakra, located at the level of the heart.

Asana: Yogic posture.

Baba: Neem Karoli Baba, Ma Jaya's beloved guru.

Bhagavati: A youthful aspect of the Mother.

Chakra: An energy center within the body, or a place where energy channels meet in a clockwise swirling pattern. There are thousands of chakras, but the seven main ones are along the spine at the places where the three main energy channels, or nadis, cross.

Chidakash: The heart space over the head, a place of compassionate detachment; also known as Sky of Consciousness or Sky Mind. This was a core teaching of Swami Bhagavan Nitynanda.

Cosmic Consciousness: Higher spiritual awareness, in which we experience that our personal consciousness is part of universal consciousness.

Ego: The small self. Identification with the ego keeps us separate from the universal self.

Ganesh: The elephant-headed god in Hinduism. Ganesh is invoked at the start of new endeavors because he brings blessings and removes obstacles.

Ganga, Ganges: Sacred river in India, considered by many to be a goddess in her own right. She is invoked as a symbol for many flowing motions, including the breath, the movement of life force up the spine, and the tantric flow of life into death, death into life.

Hanuman: The Hindu god of service; an incarnation of Lord Shiva who came to earth in the form of a monkey to teach us humility.

Ida: Energy channel on the left side, representing the feminine, coolness, and the moon.

Kapalabhati, Kabalabathi: A breath practice involving powerful contractions of the belly to create a series of strong exhalations.

Kali: The dark goddess Kali, though terrifying in appearance, assists those on the spiritual path by consuming their impurities and karma.

Kali Natha Yoga, Kali Natha Kundalini Tantric Yoga: Ancient yoga handed down from Lord Shiva through the lineage of the Nathas and given to us by Ma Jaya.

Karma: The universal law of cause and effect. Karma manifests in our lives as patterns of thought and action that seem to control us. However, freedom is always available.

Kundalini, Kundalini Shakti: The transformative goddess energy that lies dormant at the base of the spine until she is awakened. She rises up the sushumna or spinal column through each of the seven main chakras. At the top of the head Shakti merges with the masculine energy, Shiva, and enters the formless.

Manipura: The third chakra, located at the solar plexus or navel.

Maya: Illusion, distraction, impermanence, the material world. Maya may be dismissed as illusion, or she may be celebrated as the manifestation of the Mother, or both.

Mother: The divine Mother, great goddess, female energy. She holds all form, all objects, all thoughts and feelings, as she dances with the formless.

Mudra: Special gesture known to yogis, which may be used in worship, healing, and prayer. The word literally means "seal," as it seals a moment in time and space.

Muladhara: The first chakra, near the base of the spine.

Mystic: One who knows, or seeks, the direct experience of divinity.

Nadi: Energy channel or meridian in the body.

Nath, Natha: An ancient lineage of spiritual masters. It is said that they handed down yoga in a direct transmission from Shiva.

Neem Karoli Baba: Ma Jaya's beloved guru, who she usually called simply "Baba." He was known throughout India by many names. He is known for his teaching "Feed Everyone."

Nityananda, Swami Bhagavan Nityananda: Ma Jaya's teacher. An Indian holy man, believed by many to have been a perfect master from birth. After traveling widely in India, he established an ashram at Ganeshpuri, and left his body in 1961.

Non-breath: When the breath stops in meditation, it is the merge of Shiva and Shakti, masculine and feminine, and the place of non-duality.

Pingala: Energy channel on the right side, representing the masculine, heat, and the sun.

Prana: The vital life force, active and alive within us; eternal, pure life energy that regulates and connects every process in the universe.

Pranam: Prayer pose, or anjali mudra, with palms together; also a common greeting or sign of respect in India.

Pranayama: Yogic breath, the science of breath control, the fourth of eight limbs in classical yoga.

Ram: The name of God in Sanskrit, the formless essence.

Ramakrishna: An Indian holy man who was a devotee of the Mother, especially in her form as Kali.

Rumi: Thirteenth century Persian poet, scholar, and Sufi mystic who often used the word "Beloved" to express his love for God.

Sacred Bone: The coccyx or tailbone, located an inch below the base of the spine. This is our primary point of spiritual contact with the earth.

Sadhana: Spiritual practices such as mantra, chanting, pranayama, yoga, and meditation.

Sadhu: Holy man, seeker, or renunciate.

Sahasrara: The chakra at the top of the head, sometimes called the 1000 petaled lotus.

Samadhi: State of enlightenment, bliss, completion, or union with God.

Samsara: The physical world, the world of illusion, and the cycle of birth and death controlled by our karma and attachments.

Samskara: Deeply rooted karmic habit pattern.

Shakti: The female power of the universe, expressed as movement, love, and joy. When merged with Shiva she becomes the essence of Shiva-Shakti, without time or space.

Shiva: God of destruction and rebirth, transformation, and stillness; the masculine energy; the third aspect of the Hindu trinity.

Sitali: A cooling and relaxing breath done with the tongue formed into a U shape.

Spiritual Heart: The spiritual heart is the center of our being, located a few inches to the right of the physical heart. It is neither the physical heart nor the heart chakra, although it is associated with both.

Sushumna: The main energy channel in the body, rising up the spinal column; the axis of the body.

Svadhisthana: The second chakra, located in the area of the genitals.

Tantra, tantric: Continuation from the original source, lifetime into lifetime; the merge of the human and the divine.

Ujaya: A breath focused at the back of the throat that helps calm the mind and body; it represents victory over the mind.

Visuddha: The fifth chakra, located at the throat.

Yogi Bhajan: A Sikh teacher, also known as the Siri Singh Sahib, who brought Kundalini Yoga to the West and established Sikh Dharma.

CPSIA information can be obtained
at www.ICGtesting.com
Printed in the USA
BVHW041152060519
547459BV00009B/939/P

9 780983 822837